THE
10-MINUTE L.E.A.P.

THE 10-MINUTE L.E.A.P.

Lifetime Exercise Adherence Plan

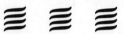

Richard L. Brown, Ph.D.

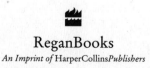

ReganBooks
An Imprint of HarperCollins*Publishers*

HarperCollins books may be purchased for educational, business, or sales promotional use. For information please write: Special Markets Department, HarperCollins Publishers, Inc., 10 East 53rd Street, New York, NY 10022.

FIRST EDITION

Designed by Interrobang Design Studio

Library of Congress Cataloging-in-Publication Data
Brown, Richard L., 1937–
    The ten minute l.e.a.p. : lifetime exercise adherence plan / Richard L. Brown.—1st ed.
        p. cm.
    Includes bibliographical references and index.
    ISBN 0–06–039249–5
    1. Exercise—Health aspects.   I. Title.
RA781.B765   1998   98-11427
613.7′1—dc21   CIP

---

97 98 99 00 01   10 9 8 7 6 5 4 3 2 1

This book is intended to help you make physical activity a part of your life. It is not intended to replace medical advice or be a substitute for a physician. Before beginning this or any physical activity program, check with your physician, especially if you have a medical problem.

To the 45 million Americans who believe in the value of fitness and have attempted exercise programs again and again, but have not yet made physical activity a consistent part of their lives. And to those who enjoy the challenge of trying to get the best from themselves.

If you can multiply 3 numbers together, you can make physical activity a consistent, enjoyable part of your life.

)))) CONTENTS ((((

WHY THE 10-MINUTE L.E.A.P.?

When you finish reading *The 10-Minute L.E.A.P.* you will have a place to begin your physical activity program that is exactly right for you. You will have solid guidelines that help you know how much activity is too little, how much is too much, and how to progress safely and consistently. You will have a powerful tool that will help you make physical activity a part of your life.

Not all of us start at the same place. We start at our own individual optimal level, and build from there.

Organizations, like the American Medical Association, the Surgeon General's Office, the American College of Sports Medicine, and the American Heart Association, have provided suggestions of frequencies (days per week), durations (minutes per workout), and intensities (how hard) that will probably result in physical benefits. Along with a safe starting level, an optimal level of physical activity, and an overtraining level, I have also incorporated those guidelines in the book. They are divided into:

Your Safe Starting Level
Your Disease Risk Reduction Level
Your Body Composition Change Level
Your Cardiovascular Improvement Level
Your Optimal Training Level
Your Overtraining Level.

Depending upon your current health and fitness your Optimal Training Level could be below the Disease Risk Reduction Level, above the Cardiovascular Improvement Level, or somewhere in between.

If you are currently inactive, the best thing for you may be simply to begin an activity program by putting 10 minutes of physical activity into your life each day. Hence, *The 10-Minute L.E.A.P.* It won't get you to the disease risk reduction level, but it is a start, is much, much better than being inactive, and it will insure you can make physical activity a part of your life.

As you become more fit you can build up to three 10-minute sessions of physical activity a day. Another 10-minute theme. Then you could progress until you are doing 30 continuous minutes a day of low intensity aerobic exercise every day or almost every day of the week. This will promote disease risk reduction benefits.

Now if you increase the intensity to a moderate level for the same 30 minutes a day for just 4 days a week, you could enjoy changes in body composition. Then if you increase the time to 40 minutes a day at moderate intensity for the same 4 days you could experience cardiovascular improvement.

Those of you who are already at or above your Cardiovascular Improvement Level could begin at Your Optimal Training Level.

There is something in L.E.A.P. for everybody. But for those of you who are currently inactive, it can all begin with a 10-Minute L.E.A.P.

Okay, put yourself in my shoes. I'm at the top of my field, a "fitness authority." I'm supposed to know more about fitness than most people. Right? So what do I do when one day a great big bear walks into my office and says, "I've got a fitness secret even you don't know."

"Who are you?" I say.

And the bear says, "I'm Dick Brown. I've coached hundreds of people. Seven of them went to the Olympics and World Championships and won two Gold Medals and three Silver Medals. I want you to help me share my secret of how I got them there."

"No one will listen," I shot back. "They don't want to go to the Olympics. What good is your secret for the average Joe?"

And then I learned the beauty of Dick Brown's secret. It fits everybody. People at every level can benefit because everyone has the same problems—when am I exercising too little and when am I exercising too much?

If I feel a cold coming on, do I still go for my run and "work it out" as some athletes recommend? If I'm one hundred pounds overweight is jogging right for me? If I haven't exercised for a while, how hard should I do it when I start again? My fitness doesn't seem to be improving. How can I measure whether it's changing? If it isn't, what can I do to make it better? When do I get to rest—and for how long?

Dick Brown has invented a way of measuring your body's response to all your daily activities, from exercise, to gardening, to housework, and even to getting a good night's sleep. His method is so accurate that even subtle innuendoes of life become valid benchmarks in the long trip to better fitness.

Don't put this book aside. Your life is in the balance.

Covert Bailey
Author of *Fit or Fat*

*F*or 35 years I have worked with people who have wanted to make physical activity a lifetime habit or reach their athletic potential. Since 1982 I have coached athletes who have worked hard to become members of our Olympic and World Championship Track & Field Teams and have been fortunate to have had seven athletes make those teams. Even for the most gifted athletes, hard, intelligent work is a requirement. Equally important, their talent has to be properly channeled so that on the appropriate days athletes are able to perform to their potential. Channeling this talent, is not unlike helping someone develop a lifelong exercise habit where getting started on the right foot often spells the difference between success and failure. This is more complex and involved than it appears because the balance between health, enthausism, and optimal performance on one hand and illness, injury, boredom, and burnout on the other is often delicate.

As a long-time student of athletic performance and physical activity, in the classroom, as a coach, and as an athlete myself, I have been fortunate to have had many exceptional mentors, an opportunity to obtain a rigorous education in the physiology of exercise, and years of practical experience working with some very talented athletes.

I've also learned the importance of viewing my athletic endeavors with a little perspective. I'm not a fanatic and, like most of us, have experienced my share of missed workout days. But I have observed what works, experienced revelations, which in retrospect seem obvious, and reflected on what being physically active means. By putting these observations, revelations, and reflections into practice, I have managed to make physical activity an enjoyable habit for myself and have helped many others do the same.

This book distills the knowledge I have acquired during my years as a coach, mentor, and researcher into a revolutionary new fitness program called L.E.A.P, *Lifetime Exercise Adherence Plan*. It is a program that will help you realize your fullest potential if you are already an athlete in training and will help you achieve, painlessly and safely, the many benefits of regular exercise if you are not.

The first section, Foundations, introduces you to the three ideas upon which L.E.A.P. is built: each of us is an individual, each of us can improve our ability to consume oxygen, and for improvement to occur we must balance the challenge of physical activity with our capacity to recover from physical activity. L.E.A.P. looks at you as an individual, establishes your ability to consume oxygen, and helps you set up a physical activity program that is right for you.

The second section, The L.E.A.P. Program, will help you determine how much physical activity is exactly right for you. It will give you a place to start, a realistic goal at which to aim, and a schedule to follow that gives you answers to the questions How often? How long? How hard?

In the third section, Fine-Tuning, I use my 35 years of experience with people at all levels of physical capacity to anticipate questions you may have and problems you may encounter. I provide tips on how to get the most from the time you spend on physical activity and show you strategies to help you get through the rough spots that anyone physically active will experience.

Finally, the Appendixes are loaded with simple tools that help you in specific areas like training schedules, diet, intensity measurements, stress reduction, and motivation. You will also find concepts relating to physical activity that I wish I had known about sooner. These may help make your physical activity more fun or help you get greater enjoyment and benefits out of your L.E.A.P. program. An extensive bibliography, from which *The 10-Minute L.E.A.P.* was partially developed, concludes the book.

The 10-Minute L.E.A.P. draws upon a constantly growing body of research on exercise and health. Scientists like Hans Selye, Thomas Cureton, Gunnar Borg, Ralph Paffenbarger, David Clarke, Jack Wilmore, David Costill, Michael Pollock, and Mel Williams have produced research that has significantly influenced me in the development of *The 10-Minute L.E.A.P.* Bill Bowerman and Arthur Lydiard are not only great coaches but also pioneers in promoting exercise for everyone. They are mentors who have helped me learn how to combine science and art, making the scientific knowledge useful to anyone who wants to improve performance or to be fit. By training in the late '60s and early '70s using Aerobic Points, an exercise system developed by Dr. Kenneth Cooper, I was introduced to the benefits that accrue from the interaction of numbers and exercise. It is upon foundations like this that L.E.A.P. is built, which help make it the most advanced exercise concept available today.

Taking into account the physics of physical activity and the careful equilibrium between challenge and recovery, L.E.A.P. helps you achieve a maximum rate of consistent improvement without fear of burnout or injury. People want physical activity to be a part of their lives. *The 10-Minute L.E.A.P.* is your key to making it a consistent, beneficial, and enjoyable part of your life.

THE
10-MINUTE L.E.A.P.

CHAPTER 1

THE 10-MINUTE L.E.A.P.,
THE POWER OF TWO NUMBERS

*P*erhaps in the future, science will discover a way for you to maintain vibrant health while you remain sedentary. But for now, the fountain of youth can only be achieved by being physically active, eating intelligently, and respecting rest.

Of these three habits, physical activity may be the most powerful because on its coattails ride good diet and respect for rest. Being active increases your incentive to eat well and rest properly; having a good diet or being good at rest does not provide the same stimulus for incorporating the other two habits into your life. Now, a revolutionary breakthrough in activity technology, named L.E.A.P., can help you experience the power of being physically active and capture the best elements of eternal youth: stamina and strength, immunity and sexual drive, curiousity and enthusiasm.

Physical activity is powerful because it strongly influences your constantly changing body. Some of these changes are dramatic, such as when you slip and must be quick enough and strong enough to catch yourself. Most changes, however, are small, unceasing, and inconspicuous. For example, these constant little changes can impede your blood or allow it to continue flowing smoothly, cause your bones to become brittle or maintain their supportive qualities, reduce your muscle strength or allow you to be strong throughout your life.

On L.E.A.P., regular physical activity will help influence the quantity and quality of your life. Being active will affect every cell, tissue, organ, and system in your body. It will keep your heart powerful and your blood flowing. It will keep your bones strong and your muscles pliable. It will keep your nerves calm and your hormones in sync. It will keep your lungs clear and your skin glowing. It will keep your cells supplied with nutrients and your body free of waste. It will keep your immunity higher and your reproductive system more potent. Because physical activity does all this, it slows aging. L.E.A.P. can help add years to your life.

But that's not the best part. The best part is that L.E.A.P. can help you, through physical activity, add life to your years. You'll feel better. Why? Because you're healthier, so you've reduced your risk of disease. You're more relaxed because you've given stress a place to go. You're better looking because you've improved your muscle-to-fat ratio. Your performance is better, vocationally, recreationally, and sexually, because you have more energy. You're more confident because you feel that energy. You like yourself better because you know that when you are active you are doing something positive for yourself.

Physical activity, like food and rest, is a potent drug that people crave. People want to be physically active. But there's a problem: Well over 45 million Americans say they believe in the benefits of physical activity, but continue to fail in their attempts to make physical activity a regular part of their lives.

Why do they fail? There are lots of excuses: lack of time, boredom, inconvenience, fatigue, nobody cares anyway, I just gain the weight back, it won't make a difference, the dog chewed my tennis shoes.

But in reality, all of these excuses boil down to two simple reasons:

1. Inertia–Things at rest tend to stay at rest.

2. Uncertainty—I don't know if what I'm doing is doing any good.

Even top athletes face these obstacles on a regular basis. Nothing illustrates this better than a quote from the great Australian runner and world record holder Ron Clarke, who when asked what was the hardest thing he had to do in training answered, "To put on me shorts and get out the door."

And for most of us, even if we get out the door, we're uncertain about what's right for us. What physical activities are best for me? How often should I do them? How long? How hard?

L.E.A.P. is an exercise solution that will help get you out the door and show you what is exactly right for you. L.E.A.P. acts as your personal fitness mentor so you can make physical activity a part of your life and realize all the benefits of exercise.

L.E.A.P.'s efficacy and power lies in two numbers that enable you to overcome inertia and eliminate uncertainty. The first number tells you how much energy your body is capable of converting. This number, your Energy Conversion Number, gives you an honest, almost medically accurate measurement of your own physiology. It tells you how successful your body is in converting energy. And it is a very personal number. It is different for everyone who follows the program, which is why L.E.A.P., unlike any other fitness concept, truly acts like a mentor who knows your abilities, goals, and needs.

Your Energy Conversion Number shows you how the exercise, as well as the nonexercise aspects of your life, influences your ability to convert energy. These nonexercise aspects include body demographics, sleep, relaxation, nutrition, support, and time available. By making certain changes in your lifestyle, changes that do not add any extra commitments to your schedule, you can make a significant positive difference in your level of health and energy conversion ability before you even put on your sweats.

From your Energy Conversion Number you can generate a second number, your Energy Conversion Points (ECPs). ECPs tell you two things:

1. How much energy you convert each time you exercise
2. How much energy you should be converting each week through physical activity in order to maintain or improve your health, fitness, and quality of life

ECPs provide goals that are specifically designed for you and give prompt feedback on your progress toward those goals. ECPs remove all the guesswork people normally experience when they commence a fitness program.

ECPs also give you unprecedented flexibility to choose and change the type, frequency, duration, and intensity of your exercise activity whenever you wish. With L.E.A.P., you don't have to stick with just a few physical activities. L.E.A.P. enables you to participate in an almost unlimited number of activities, including physical labor, and encourages you to try as many as you want. Trying different activities increases your chances of finding activities that are fun. And more than anything else, fun is a big lever when it comes to overcoming inertia. Finally, ECPs give you an exact way to chart your progress as you approach your goal.

ECPs define upper limits of energy conversion so that you can avoid getting sick or injured as a result of overtraining. ECPs show you the value of all activities, those that everyone says are exercise and those that many say are not really exercise, like gardening or vacuuming the house. ECPs even allow you to turn the evaluation process around and play "What if. . . ?" so that you can plan workouts specific to your needs for the day or the week. For example, what if I want to score 35 ECPs riding a bike but only have 20 minutes to ride, how hard should I ride? For novice to serious athletes, this potentiates the ability to stay healthy, make progress, and make physical performance a part of life.

L.E.A.P. helps you gauge your current capabilities. Then it shows you where to start your exercise program and how to pick goals you can achieve. L.E.A.P. guides you toward those goals, keeping challenge and recovery balanced. L.E.A.P. enables you to measure your progress toward each goal and accurately evaluate what you have done every time you are active. And L.E.A.P. is simple. If you can multiply 3 numbers together you can do L.E.A.P. and make physical activity an enjoyable part of your life.

Intelligent physical activity is the drug for longevity, quality of life, and physical independence. L.E.A.P. is the prescription.

PART 1

FOUNDATIONS

The following three chapters explain the science and theory behind L.E.A.P., illustrating in detail why the program is so effective. But if you are eager to plunge right in and begin learning how to use L.E.A.P., feel free to skip ahead to Part 2.

L.E.A.P. is based on three fundamental concepts: individuality, VO_2Max, and Hans Selye's General Adaptation syndrome. The first, individuality, represents the sum of the characteristics that set you apart from everybody else. The second, VO_2Max, is the maximum amount of oxygen you can consume at any time. The third, Hans Selye's General Adaptation syndrome, is perhaps the most important training concept ever proposed.

CHAPTER 2

INDIVIDUALITY

*I*ndividuality has to be respected. Each of us is unique. If our feet are size 7, we don't do very well wearing size 5 or size 9 shoes. Similarly, individuality must be the cornerstone of any physical activity program. While many fitness facilities pay lip service to individuality, they often fail to follow through on their claims. Why is that? Without understanding each individual's ability to convert[1] energy and the factors that contribute to that ability, it is difficult to develop an effective physical activity program for an individual.

Furthermore, without a consistent method for estimating energy conversion, it is difficult to determine how much energy you need to convert for improvement, how much energy you have already converted in a workout, or how much energy you have left to convert.

Another problem with fitness programs is that they usually are either very general or involve significant personal supervision. Those that tend to generalize create a situation where the activities are too difficult for some people. These people drop out or get hurt. If the program is too easy, little benefit is derived from following it.

On the other hand, those that involve constant, effective supervision are expensive. People who are true fitness mentors have years of education and experience and as a result

---

[1]I use the words *convert energy* throughout the book where other authors might use *expend*. Either term is acceptable. I prefer *convert* because energy can be neither created nor destroyed. Energy can only be converted from one form to another.

are able to demand a high premium just like other valued health professionals. But a situation of constant, effective supervision is rare. People can't afford it, don't understand how valuable it can be if they truly need it, and there are relatively few knowledgeable, experienced professionals.

Too many people in the supervisory capacity are simply not qualified. Just because someone is strong, young, or can run fast doesn't mean they know how to advise you as an individual. Too often their advice is based upon "this is what works for me." Often fitness employees are people who are hired at minimum wages by clubs to encourage and push clients. Even if they have "credentials" it may mean very little. You can get credentials to be a fitness advisor in just 3 months by buying a recommended text, paying a testing fee, and passing a test based on that text. Would you want the dentist working on your teeth to have earned credentials that way?

Even if the supervisors are qualified, a lot of things can still go wrong. I was in an expensive health club on the East Coast a few years ago. I watched as each member turned in a workout card to the fitness advisor by placing it in a basket on his desk. The basket was overflowing with cards. "You never look at those, do you?" I asked. "I don't have the time," he replied. How was he going to give accurate and honest feedback to his clients? How was he going to gain a true understanding of how much energy these individuals could safely and intelligently convert?

There are, to be sure, clubs and personal trainers that are doing great work. Some personal trainers I know don't have a formal education, but they have a great affection for physical activity and people. This motivates them to learn and helps them get it right. They are like the teacher we may all remember that volunteered to coach a sport nobody else wanted and who ended up not only caring for the sport and the students, but also becoming a very good coach, despite the low stipend for the time spent. These people succeed because they truly care about you as an individual.

Because the cornerstone of L.E.A.P. is its ability to help you understand and respect your personal ability to convert energy, you get the same service that only the best mentors can provide. L.E.A.P. is able to treat you as an individual, and individuality is the foundation for any physical activity program.

What exactly does treating yourself as an individual mean? First, forget for a few minutes about age, gender, weight, and the many other factors that are extremely relevant. We'll come back to them in Part 2. For now, think of the basic underlying individual characteristic that really determines what is physically right for you. That characteristic is your ability to convert energy. How much energy can you safely and intelligently convert through physical activity?

In setting up any physical activity program, from cardiac rehabilitation to Olympic training, the ability to convert energy determines everything else in the program: where you start, how much you do, how hard you do it, how often you do it, and how you progress. When you finish Part 2, you will know how much energy you can convert and what that means for you in terms of a physical activity program. But first, what do I mean when I use the term *energy*?

WHAT IS ENERGY?

Energy is the ability to do work. Energy can be potential energy or kinetic energy. Potential energy is stored, waiting to be used, like the energy in the chemical bonds of a glucose or adenosine triphosphate (ATP) molecule. Kinetic energy is the energy of motion, like the energy of muscles contracting.

Energy comes in various forms. There is thermal energy, which is the energy of the movement of the atoms in a substance. The faster the movement, the hotter the substance.

There is chemical energy, which is the energy released from the bonds that hold molecules together. There is electrical energy, which is the energy of electron movement in substances that conduct electricity. There is mechanical energy, which is the energy of a mass in motion.

The Law of Conservation of Energy states that energy is conserved; it can be neither created nor destroyed but only be changed in form. Energy is continually converted from one form to another. For example, two results occur when the bond between the second and third phosphate in ATP is broken in a muscle cell: energy is converted from chemical energy to thermal energy and to mechanical energy. The temperature rises, and a muscle contracts. When the muscles contract we can move, and we might move a rock to the top of a table. When the rock is resting at that height above the ground, the energy has been converted to potential energy.

Living things require a constant flow of energy. Plants convert radiant energy from the sun to chemical energy in carbohydrates. The animals that eat the plants convert the energy in the chemical bonds to empower functions that maintain life. These processes convert a significant portion of the energy to heat, which is returned to the environment. Living things must devote a considerable portion of their structure to acquiring and converting energy.[2]

Energy really is everything. Even though we see many things around us every day, all there is in the universe is energy. It is true that this energy can be converted to mass— everything we sense—but ultimately everything is energy. Einstein's formula $E = mc^2$[3] shows that energy and mass are interchangeable.

---

[2] One scientific unit of energy is the joule. One joule is equal to 1 kg x m^2/sec^2. There are approximately 4.2 joules in 1 calorie. When we consume 1 liter of oxygen, we convert approximately 4.85 calories of energy.

[3] E = energy, m = mass, c = speed of light.

WHY SHOULD I KNOW ABOUT ENERGY?

Although we usually don't think of laws of physics as directly concerning us, two laws of physics demonstrate the importance of energy in our everyday lives. The first, the Law of Conservation of Energy, as previously mentioned, states that energy can neither be created nor destroyed, only changed from one form to another.

This law forms the basis for energy flow in all living things and lies at the heart of one of industrial societies' major problems and fixations, fat. This is the scenario:

1. In industrial countries, food (energy) is abundant.
2. The food is often high in calories and low in nutritional value.
3. People engulf more food than they can use because industrial societies advertise nutrient-free foods and promote a sedentary lifestyle.
4. Since energy cannot be destroyed, excess energy is converted to fat, an energy warehouse.

The basic reality for one-third of the population in the United States can be described by the following formula:

Too Much Energy In + Not Enough Energy Converted to Work/Heat = Too Much Energy Stored as Fat

There's no way around this physical law. If you take in more energy than you convert for metabolic requirements, you will convert the remaining energy to be stored as fat. As can easily be observed at any mall or fast food franchise where customers belly up to the counter, store it we have. Even more frightening, the same phenomenon can be observed in our schools, where the children are fatter and more sedentary than at any time in our history. Fat drives much of corporate America, where billions upon billions of dollars are spent trying to get us to ignore the Law of Conservation of Energy and then spent again treating the result of our inattention to that law.

It is becoming more normal, but not more healthy, in the United States for energy balance to be out of balance. Even if this imbalance is only 350 calories per week (a slice of cake once a week), after 10 weeks a person has gained a pound of fat (3,500 calories equate to a pound of fat). After a year, the same person will have gained 5 pounds. In five years, seemingly out of nowhere, that person is 25 pounds heavier.

But you can have your cake and eat it too, by becoming physically active as opposed to sedentary. By converting more energy through physical activity, you insure that less is stored as fat. Only 60 minutes of gardening, walking, or golfing, 35 minutes of jogging, cycling, or swimming, or 90 minutes of milking by hand will be enough to change the energy in the slice of cake from energy stored to energy converted, and that's something to get excited about.

There is another physical law that has everyday ramifications in our lives—the Second Law of Thermodynamics. It states that energy must continually flow through a system to keep it intact, or the system will degenerate.

Energy always flows from a higher level to a lower level. Pour warm soup into a cool bowl. If left alone, the soup will heat the bowl until the soup and the bowl are at the same temperature. When they are at the same temperature, energy flow ceases. It is then said that the entropy of the system has been reached.

Entropy is the name given to energy that has gone from available energy to unavailable energy. Entropy, or unavailable energy, is continuously increasing in the universe because energy is continually flowing from a higher level to a lower level.

Where our solar system and life on earth are concerned, the Second Law of Thermodynamics gives us the end of the story. When the energy of the sun runs out, there will be no light, and all energy flow will cease. $E = mc^2$. When $c = 0$, then $E = 0$. With no sun, energy levels in our solar system will all be equal, and energy can no longer be converted. All energy will then be entropy or unavailable energy. However, the death of the sun is not very meaningful, because the sun can produce energy for another 5 billion years.

What is meaningful to us is that if energy is not continuously converted to maintain our bodies, our bodies also will degenerate. So if you want to be a healthy, fully functioning individual, your body must have the ability to efficiently convert energy.

We pay a grave price for our inattention to the Second Law of Thermodynamics. Degenerative diseases are an example of what occurs when energy becomes entropy. Muscle tissue wastes away, leaving us more vulnerable to injuries when we are required to do something physical. Bones break more easily because they become more brittle. The heart must work harder to pump blood because the walls of the arteries lose their elasticity and become clogged with fat. Cells don't get as much blood because the number of capillaries going past them is reduced. The cell can't convert as much energy because the mitochondrial protein, the cell's power plant, is reduced. These are just a few of the effects of not maintaining efficient energy flow through the body that result in the epidemic of degenerative diseases affecting industrial societies today. And as with the Law of Conservation of Energy, whether we like the implications or not, we are bound by this inescapable law of nature.

I recently realized how several common sayings illustrate the dilemmas of thermodynamics in an intriguing fashion. Consider:

"You can't fight the system!" You have no choice: Your body will obey natural laws whether you like it or not.

"You can't get something for nothing!" You've got to keep energy flowing or your account will soon be empty.

"You're up the creek without a paddle!" You've stopped supplying energy effectively and are now at the mercy of the entropy current.

"There's no use crying over spilt milk!" When energy has become entropy, you can't get it back.

Ultimately, we are all defined as individuals by our ability to convert energy. L.E.A.P. is a powerful tool enabling you to maintain the energy flow instead of storing it and to oppose entropy by making your body's energy conversions more efficient.

CHAPTER 3

VO$_2$MAX

*E*ach person's ability to convert energy is unique. How do you determine what level of energy conversion via physical activity is right for you? It turns out that the amount of oxygen your cells can consume is an excellent measure of your ability to convert energy, and this amount is one of the foundations L.E.A.P. uses to construct a program tailored just for you. The symbol for the most oxygen you can use is VO$_2$Max. VO$_2$Max is a benchmark that is used worldwide as a valid measure of physical fitness.

> V = volume
> O$_2$ = oxygen
> Max = maximum (the most)

VO$_2$Max represents the most oxygen you can consume. It is measured in milliliters of oxygen per kilogram of body weight per minute.

VO$_2$Max units = ml/kg/min

If you have a VO$_2$Max of 45, it means that the most oxygen you can convert is 45 ml for every kilogram of your body weight for every minute you are active. If you weighed 65 kg and were active for 1 minute, the most oxygen you could use during that time would be 2925 ml.

> Oxygen Used = VO$_2$Max x Weight x Time
> Oxygen Used = 45 ml x 65 x 1 = 2925 ml[1]

But L.E.A.P. doesn't require you to go out and get your VO2Max measured. Instead, by answering simple questions about your lifestyle and applying the formulas derived and modified from L.E.A.P.'s computer program to your answers, it is possible to determine your VO2Max safely, accurately, and absolutely painlessly.

Whenever I commit to work with anyone, Olympic athlete or cardiac rehabilitation patient, the first characteristic I determine is their VO2Max. The ability to use oxygen is directly related to how much energy you can convert. It defines you as an individual. I know that if I give you guidelines based on your ability to convert energy, and you stay within those guidelines, you will be able to train safely, intelligently, and consistently, enhancing your ability to perform on cue or to reach your fitness goals.

It has been determined that at rest humans consume about 3.5 ml/kg/min of oxygen. Someone who is not able to expend much energy in physical activity, who gets winded going to the mailbox, might have a VO2Max of 20 ml/kg/min. The highest VO2Max in humans is somewhere around 80 ml/kg/min of oxygen. Someone who can expend energy very well, who can run forever, might have a VO2Max of 80 ml/kg/min. This means the second person has an "oxygen well" (the quantity of oxygen the body can draw upon) almost five times deeper than that of the first.

$$\text{Oxygen Well}_{20} = 20 - 3.5 = 16.5 \text{ ml/kg/min}$$
$$\text{Oxygen Well}_{80} = 80 - 3.5 = 76.5 \text{ ml/kg/min}$$

---

[1] A soft drink can has a volume of 350 ml, so a 65-kg person with a VO2Max of 45 could consume 8.4 soft drink cans filled with oxygen in 1 minute when they were working as hard as he/she could. Soft Drink Cans = 2925 ÷ 350 /can = 8.4 Cans

Difference in Oxygen Available = 76.5 − 16.5 = 60 ml/kg/min

' Difference in Depth of Oxygen Well = 76.5 ÷ 16.5 = 4.6

Since oxygen enables chemical bonds originating in food substances to be converted to other types of energy, the person with a VO2Max of 80 has a much better energy conversion ability.

Table 3.1 compares these two people to show the difference VO2Max can make in completing a physical activity. For the example, let's assume that both people are running as hard as they can. The person with a VO2Max of 20 can run a little more than .6 miles in 10 minutes. The person with a VO2Max of 80 can cover almost 2.5 miles in 10 minutes.

Table 3.1

	VO2Max = 20	VO2Max = 80
Oxygen Consumed (liters)	13	52
Energy Converted (calories)	63	252
Work Done (miles)	.62	2.40

Energy Conversion Comparison

In this book, examples are often presented along with the math. The math is included so that you can understand how a result was calculated. You can always skip the math. It won't change the point I am trying to make in the example.

The physical activity for both = 10-minute run
The body weight of both = 65 kg (143 lb)
The VO2Max of Person 1 = 20 ml/kg/min
The VO2Max of Person 2 = 80 ml/kg/min

Person 1 can use 13,000 ml of oxygen in the 10 minutes.

20 ml/kg/min x 65kg x 10 min = 13 liters

Person 2 can use 52,000 ml of oxygen in the 10 minutes.

80 ml/kg/min x 65kg x 10 min = 52 liters

It takes 1 liter of oxygen to convert 4.85 calories of energy.
Person 1 is able to convert 63 calories.

13 liters x 4.85 cal/liter = 63 cal

Person 2 is able to convert 260 calories.

52 liters x 4.85 cal/liter = 252 cal

If you weigh 65 kg, it takes about 105 calories to travel 1 mile.
Person 1 can travel about .60 miles in 10 minutes.

63 /105 per mile = .60 miles

Person 2 can travel about 2.40 miles in 10 minutes.

252 /105 per mile = 2.40 miles[3]

From the example you can see that the person with the higher VO_2Max is:

---

[3] The current world record for 2 miles is just under 4 min/mile, and the current world record for 5000 meters (3.1 miles) is a little over 4 min/mile.

1. Able to go farther
2. Because more energy is converted
3. When more oxygen is used

The ability to use oxygen affects all aspects of your life because you must continually supply oxygen to the cells of your body so that they can continually convert energy. You will rarely work at your maximum ability to use oxygen, nor should you. Working at your maximum ability to convert energy is very expensive physically and demands total emotional involvement.

But you will always be working at some percentage of your maximum. For example, if a landscaping job required 18 ml/kg/min of oxygen, the person with the VO2Max of 20 would be working at 90% of VO2Max while the person with the VO2Max of 80 would be working at only 22% of VO2Max. The first person would find the work more intense and would need much more recovery time after the job was completed. As you will learn, in the L.E.A.P. program you will measure your intensity by understanding at what percentage of your VO2Max you are working.

Using a real-life example, let me illustrate the point that you are always converting energy at some percentage of your VO2Max. Marlene, the lady with whom I live, weighs 65 kg and has a VO2Max of 45 ml/kg/min. If it takes 3.5 ml/kg/min to live, she is always consuming about 7.8% of her VO2Max to stay alive.

$$3.5 \div 45 = .078 = 7.8\%$$

Now, pretend we hook Marlene up to an instrument that measures how much oxygen she consumes while working in the garden, which she loves to do. She works in the garden for 30 minutes, and when she is finished we find that she used 46,800 ml of oxygen. Since the most she could use in

30 minutes would be 87,750 ml, it means that she was working at 53% of her VO_2Max.

O$_2$ Used at 100% VO_2Max = 45 ml/kg/min x 65kg x 35 min = 87,750 ml
  46,800 ÷ 87,750 = .53 = 53% of VO_2Max

Since 1000 ml of oxygen converts approximately 4.85 calories of energy, it means that as Marlene consumed 46,800 ml of oxygen she converted 227 calories of energy in her gardening effort. It doesn't seem like much, but calories accumulate quickly. If Marlene did the same amount of gardening 3 days a week for a year, she would convert slightly over 35,000 calories. That's the equivalent of about 10 pounds of fat. Just by converting energy doing the gardening, which may not seem like exercise at all, she's not storing the energy in 10 pounds of fat. That's another reason for L.E.A.P.'s efficacy. L.E.A.P. recognizes that everyday activities that increase oxygen consumption convert energy and really do count as exercise.

HOW DOES L.E.A.P. ESTIMATE VO$_2$MAX?

In Part 2 you will get an estimate of your VO_2Max by answering questions about aspects of your life that affect your ability to deliver and use oxygen. These aspects of your life include age, gender, fat-free weight, sleep, relaxation, nutrition, support, time, and current physical activity. While you can always ask a physician or laboratory to do a VO_2 test, I have rarely determined VO_2Max in this manner. The tests are expensive, very dependent upon the calibration of the equipment and the experience of the technician, and they often require a maximal effort.

Physical tests are not required, because it has been shown that biographical estimates are accurate and correlate well with laboratory data. I have been using the questions you will be asked for over 10 years and have found the VO2Max estimated by the interview to be consistent and reliable. It is not unusual for someone to do the interview and then comment that they recently took a lab VO2Max test and that the results of the interview are within a few milliliters of the results of the test.

In 1990 the results of a 2000-person study done by NASA and the University of Houston, "Prediction of Functional Aerobic Capacity without Exercise Testing," were published in *Medicine and Science in Sports and Exercise*. The authors of the article came to the conclusion that their procedure for predicting VO2Max without exercise testing was "more accurate than established submaximal treadmill tests and appropriate for 96% of the adult population."

To see how the L.E.A.P. autobiography and prediction formula compared with those in the NASA/Houston test, I took 25 people whose VO2Max I knew and asked them the questions from both the NASA/Houston test and L.E.A.P.. Between VO2Max 30 and 60, the results were almost identical. Below a VO2Max of 30 and above a VO2Max of 60, the results from L.E.A.P. did not agree with the results of the NASA/Houston study, but it turned out that the results from L.E.A.P. in those ranges were more accurate. This was because the NASA/Houston study used linear regression to develop their predictions and L.E.A.P. used power regression. Power regression formulas account for curves in the regression line, while in linear regression all predictions occur around a straight line. The NASA/Houston authors made this additional comment about their study: "the accuracy of the predictions was upheld with all but subjects with a VO2Peak > 55 ml/kg/min." L.E.A.P.'s estimate of VO2Max from the autobiography in Part 2 is based in large part upon L.E.A.P.'s power regression formulas and can be used with confidence.

HOW DOES L.E.A.P. USE VO2MAX?

When you have an estimate of your VO2Max, what can you do with it? L.E.A.P. uses VO2Max in five ways:

1. To determine an energy conversion starting point that is right for you
2. To establish a range of energy conversions in which you will experience various degrees of success: a safe minimum level, a disease risk reduction level, a body composition change level, a cardiovascular improvement level, an optimal level, an overtraining level
3. To set up a 13-week program that will allow you to progress in such a way that physical adaptation occurs, improving your ability to convert energy
4. To measure your progress
5. To determine intensities of effort that will be safe for you

Each of these points will be explained in more detail in other parts of the book. But now let's talk about how L.E.A.P. uses VO2Max to determine intensity of effort—how hard you're working.

PERCEIVED EXERTION

Being introduced to L.E.A.P.'s use of VO2Max to determine how hard you're working will help you understand how percentage of VO2Max is a central theme of physical activity and of the L.E.A.P. program.

Physical activities can be divided into two intensity classifications: pace activities and nonpace activities. The intensity of pace activities can be determined by a time-to-distance ratio. Running, walking, swimming, and cycling are examples of pace activities. To get an intensity, or pace, you simply divide the time by the distance. If you ran 2 miles in 22 minutes, your pace would be 11 minutes per mile.

Pace can be used to determine at what percentage of VO2Max you are working, and VO2Max can be used to determine what paces are right for you. However, it is difficult to determine paces for different individuals seeking different goals, working out at different distances on different days in a variety of environmental conditions. Determining these paces using all the variables, including VO2Max, can be done, but it requires some degree of physiological sophistication and the aid of a computer.

In addition, there are many physical activities that do not have a distance component. Most of the 150 activities on the L.E.A.P. Activity List (which you will learn about later) are nonpace activities. Court sports, racquet sports, aerobics, downhill skiing, housework, and gardening are examples of activities that do not have a distance component so that intensity cannot be determined by pace.

Can you without knowing pace, or when doing a nonpace activity, determine how hard you are working with some degree of accuracy?

There are two ways to determine intensity in these situations: heart rate and rating of perceived exertion. Heart rate may not be as simple as it sounds. You can find out more about using heart rate as a measure of intensity in Appendix D.

Rating of perceived exertion (RPE), developed by Dr. Gunnar Borg in the late 1960s, can be used by almost everyone. Borg knew that in the lab he could determine intensity by measuring oxygen consumed while people were working on special exercise equipment connected to sophisticated measuring devices. He wondered if people could accurately estimate their level of workout intensity on their own without special equipment.

He did the following experiment. While people were exercising on various pieces of equipment and while he was measuring their exercise intensity, he asked them to pick numbers and words from a chart that described how they were feeling. It turned out that the relationship between what they felt and the measured intensity was very close. Borg determined that the correlation was near 0.90. Practically, this meant that most people could accurately assess their intensity level. Dr. Borg comments on his belief in the validity of RPE:

> In my opinion, perceived exertion is the single best indicator of the degree of physical strain. The overall perceived exertion rating integrates various information, including the many signals elicited from the peripheral working muscles and joints, from the central cardiovascular and respiratory functions, and from the central nervous system. All these signals, perceptions, and experiences are integrated into a configuration of perceived exertion.

Dr. Michael Pollock, who has worked extensively with perceived exertion, backs up what Dr. Borg found:

> Even though the scale is psychological, it has a lot of physiological meaning. There is a very strong correlation between the perceptions of difficulty and actual laboratory measurement of pulse, oxygen cost, lactic acid development, and pulmonary ventilation during activity.

That the scale works so well is fortunate because it means that intensity can be judged in the field without equipment, as well as measured in the lab with equipment. Dr. Borg's rating scales are used worldwide. You can go into almost any health club and find one of the two versions of the Borg Scale of Perceived Exertion hanging on a wall.

The more recent version is called the Borg-Noble Category

Ratio Scale of Perceived Exertion. It is a scale based upon numbers and verbal expressions. Dr. Borg said, "The main idea is that numbers should be anchored by verbal expressions that are simple and understandable by people." L.E.A.P. has modified this scale by adding physiological clues to go along with the numbers and verbal expressions. In addition, L.E.A.P. has correlated percentages of VO2Max with these numbers and expressions. Finally, L.E.A.P. has developed Intensity Coefficients (Icoef) that you will use when you determine your intensity level. The Intensity Coefficients are derived from the exponential nature of increasing intensity.

All this is background. All you need to do when you are rating your activity is find your perceived exertion level on the scale and use the matching Intensity Coefficient (Icoef) in determining the amount of energy you converted.

The L.E.A.P. Modified Borg-Noble Intensity Scale is shown in Table 3.2.

Ratings of perceived exertion are easy to use. Here is a summary of some guidelines Dr. Borg provided to people in his studies:

1. During exercise, rate your perception of exertion.
2. Rate that feeling as honestly as possible. Some people want to be "brave" and rate too low. Try your best to rate your exertion as you perceive it.
3. Don't consider the exercise goal or the size of the task. The only thing of interest is your own feeling of effort and exertion.

I will add one more instruction:
4. If you are doing an intermittent activity, such as weight lifting, average the overall intensity. While you are lifting, your intensity might be very high; between lifts, your intensity will usually be lower. Try to determine an accurate average of the overall intensity of the session.

Table 3.2

RPE	Challenge was	Breathing was	Talking was	%VO2Max	ICoef
1.0	Very Easy	Normal	Normal	35	0.08
1.5				40	0.16
2.0	Easy	Normal	Normal	45	0.26
2.5				50	0.37
3.0	Moderate	Comfortable	Easy	55	0.51
3.5				60	0.66
4.0	Somewhat Strong	Noticeable	Somewhat Difficult	65	0.82
4.5				70	1.00
5.0	Strong	Deep, but Steady	Difficult	75	1.20
5.5				80	1.40
6.0	Between Strong & Very Strong	Deep & Somewhat Rapid	Between Difficult & Very Difficult	85	1.62
6.5				87.5	1.86
7.0	Very Strong	Deep & Rapid	Very Difficult	90	2.10
7.5				92.5	2.36
8.0	Very, Very Strong	Very Deep & Very Rapid	Extremely Difficult	95	2.63
8.5				96.1	2.91
9.0				97.5	3.21
9.5				98.8	3.51
10	Maximum Effort	Breathlessness	Impossible	100	3.83

Modified Borg-Noble Intensity Scale

The Modified Borg-Noble Intensity Scale also shows how %VO2Max coincides with a shift in the physiological responses of the body.

At 55% VO2Max your body is beginning to get a pronounced benefit from physical activity. At this level your exertion will feel well within your control but will begin to become noticeable. You will not notice much of a change in your breathing pattern and will easily be able to talk with a companion who might be doing the physical activity with you.

At 65% VO2Max cardiorespiratory benefits are beginning to become significant, and you will sense that you are putting forth some effort. However, you should still feel fine, and continuing at this pace should pose no problems. Your breathing will also be noticeable, and talking will be somewhat harder.

At 75% VO2Max you are in a zone where you could continue for a long period of time if you had to, but effort is getting strong, breathing is getting deep, and talking is getting hard.

At 85% VO2Max you are somewhere near the edge of steady state work. Up to this point your heart rate, breathing rate, and lactate production have risen steadily, but you sense that if you worked much harder, physiological functions would experience a sharp increase. This inflection point occurs when you are near the end of your ability to convert energy from oxygen consumption alone. The exertion is definitely strong, breathing is deep and strong, and talking is difficult.

At 90% VO2Max you are in a zone where your body has to work very hard to keep the environment of the cell stable. Oxygen use cannot meet the total demand for energy. Conversion of energy without the use of oxygen is playing a larger role, and this is an expensive way for the body to meet energy requirements because now the environment inside and outside the cells is becoming more acidic. You can keep going, but you have to push yourself very hard. Your exertion is very strong, your breathing is now deep and rapid, and you don't want to talk.

You should not feel that you must work at the higher levels of VO2Max. All physical activities are beneficial. Working at an intensity around 70% to 75% VO2Max may be very efficient, but it is not essential. You can compensate for working at a lower intensity level by working a little longer or a little more often. High intensity is sometimes required in the training program of an athlete wishing to compete at a high level, but it is not necessary for those who simply want to make physical activity a part of their life. Working at the lower end of the Modified Borg-Noble Intensity Scale usually produces fewer injuries and fewer dropouts and still produces fitness improvements. It is best to work at energy conversion and intensity levels that are appropriate for you.

In 1985, when I started working with Shelly Steely, who eventually finished 7th in the 1992 Barcelona Olympics in the women's 3000-meter run, she was only able to work for 250 minutes per week at an average of 70% of her VO_2Max, which at that time was about 64.5 ml/kg/min. By the time she was ready to run in the '92 Olympics she was working for 490 minutes per week at an average of 84% of her VO_2Max, which was then up to 68.5 ml/kg/min. It takes that type of a weekly effort to run in world-class competition. But if I had requested that she do that from the start, this is what would have happened. She may have had a reasonable first year, but she would soon have broken down and never realized her potential. Shelly is a good example of what starting at the right level of energy conversion and intensity, and then patiently developing the ability to work harder and longer, can produce.

It is important to understand that without having an accurate estimate of VO_2Max and knowing how to use it, developing an individual physical activity program for anyone would be very difficult.

CHAPTER 4

HANS SELYE'S GENERAL ADAPTATION SYNDROME

*T*he single most important foundation upon which L.E.A.P. is built is Han Selye's theory of the General Adaptation Syndrome. If you know nothing more than "in order to improve, you must balance challenge with recovery," you have far more tools in your chest than many coaches, trainers, and physicians. Each time I go to a meeting and ask, "Who is Hans Selye?" very few hands are raised. Some people understand that balancing challenge with recovery is important, but they often fail to see why.

If they knew of Selye's work they would understand the why much better. At certain points in our training, and I use the word *training* specifically because we are all athletes at one level or another, we will feel that if we work harder we will improve faster. Perhaps our results are not as good as we'd like, we're not losing weight as fast as we'd like, we have a big contest approaching, or we are not practicing very well. Most people think, erroneously, that the only answer is to work harder. If they knew Selye's theories they would know that in many cases the only logical thing to do is rest. I have seen many more outstanding performances come after rest than I have observed after someone overworks. Selye's theory addresses the need to balance challenge with recovery.

Selye first began to develop his theory when he attempted to understand why so many diseases were marked by the same basic set of symptoms: coated tongues, sore throats, achy joints, gastrointestinal disturbances, loss of appetite, loss of weight, elimination of excess amounts of nitrogen, potassium, and phosphorus, low-grade fever, enlarged spleens, and occasional rashes.

Doing research in his specialty, endocrinology, Selye saw that any extract foreign to the body produced a set of general symptoms similar to the ones he had seen in diseased patients.

At this point Selye decided that pursuing the mechanics of "just being sick" might be important in order to find out:

1. What this condition meant to an organism
2. If treatment of the nonspecific symptoms of illness was important or possible
3. If the mechanisms by which the human organism defended itself against challenges of various kinds could be improved upon
4. If some of these symptoms could be prevented

So from 1935 on, Selye devoted himself to the study of challenges to homeostasis. *Homeostasis* means staying the same. In our body's case it means keeping the environment in and around each cell compatible with cell function. Energy has to be converted and resources have to be used to accomplish homeostasis.

Selye's observations are of special importance today when stressful situations are commonplace. Indeed, he is often referred to as the Father of Stress Research. Understanding these observations is essential in developing realistic programs for sports performance and physical activity because they elegantly demonstrate the need for balance in a program, a need too often ignored today.

He observed that people seldom die of old age. They usually die of uneven wear, meaning that one system or organ gives out before the others.

He theorized that people are born with a specific amount of energy available to meet the challenges they face. This "adaptation energy" cannot be increased but can be invested wisely.

He noted that there is a ratio of local stress to total stress. If the ratio is greater than one (> 1), indicating a predominance of local stress, it suggests uneven wear on a local organ or system. If the ratio is less than one (< 1), total stress predominates, meaning that stress is spread over the body, producing even wear.

He suggested that exercise helps invest the "adaptation energy" wisely by spreading the stress more evenly over the entire body. He also suggested that being physically active stimulates a "cross-resistance," which enables the individual to meet intellectual and emotional, as well as physical, challenges.

Using these observations, Selye studied the sequence of events that occur in the body when it is faced with a challenge or challenges. Whatever one chooses to call the challenge (Selye preferred the term *stressor*), it is "a stimuli that places a demand on an organism which requires a response from that organism in order to reestablish homeostasis."

Selye found that the challenge could come in many forms: effort, fatigue, pain, fear, concentration, censure, cold, heat, exercise, starvation, infection, drugs, and a host of others, including joy, exhilaration, and success. The demand did not have to be negative; it just had to be a challenge to internal balance.

Not only can positive and negative events be viewed as challenges, but the conditions that surround the challenges can mediate their effect on the organism. The same event may elicit a different response from different people, or a different response from the same person at different times. In other words, we all look at things through the glasses of our experience, and some days are better than others.

Many challenges should not and cannot be avoided. After all, we improve by being challenged. But how many challenges we deal with and how we perceive and handle challenges are crucial to our performance and, more important, to our health and well-being.

Selye observed that the response to challenge was a sequence of adaptations made by the body as it resisted the potential damage of the challenge while maintaining homeostasis. If the challenge occurred once, an organism would either resist it or die. But if an organism was exposed repeatedly to a challenge, the response occurred in three distinct stages. The stages were the alarm stage, the adaptation stage, and the exhaustion stage. Selye called this sequence of responses the General Adaptation Syndrome. This work on alarm, adaptation, and exhaustion anchors the single most important concept for modern living and physical training: *Challenge and recovery must be balanced.*

ALARM STAGE

Physical activity above 60% VO_{2Max} triggers the "fight or flight" response, and that triggers the reactions that define the first part of the alarm stage. In the first part of this stage, the nervous and endocrine systems release their hormonal messengers, stimulating a prompt activation of resources to respond to the challenge of physical activity. Table 4.1 shows some of the changes that occur during the alarm stage as our body prepares for action.

Table 4.1

Respiration Rate Increases
Heart Rate Increases
Contractile Strength of Heart Increases
Blood Pressure Increases
Blood Flow Diverted to Muscles
Protein Broken Down to Amino Acids
Glucose Made in Liver from Amino Acids
Additional Adrenalin Produced
Glucose, Fatty Acid, Amino Acid Metabolic Rate Increases
Temperature Rises
Strength of Muscle Contraction Increases
Speed of Muscle Contraction Increases
Mental Activity Increases
Pupils Dilate
Sphincters Close

Response to Alarm

Even though physical activity may last only a small portion of the 24-hour day, the alarm stage in a well-planned physical activity program will last 24 to 48 hours. The reason it lasts longer than the activity is that, as Selye observed, based on the duration and intensity of the challenge, it takes between 24 and 48 hours to restore the resources of the body to prechallenge levels. This also implies that if an organism is not given enough time to recover from the challenge, the second time a challenge occurs the organism will not have as many resources available to meet the challenge as it had the first time.

Selye observed what happened to his laboratory animals when they entered the alarm stage. First, he saw changes in the adrenal glands. The whole adrenal gland increased in size and was embedded in a translucent layer of watery tissue. In the inner part of the adrenal gland, there was a buildup of fatty material and the appearance of empty spaces with some evidence of dead tissue in very severe stress situations. He saw in the outer part of the adrenal gland what he considered the most important adjustment in the acute defensive reaction: a dramatic increase in the production of the hormone cortisol.

Second, he observed a degenerative change in the lymphatic system. After the challenge had passed, he was able to observe debris from cells of the lymphatic system being removed by phagocytes, edema in the connective tissue, and cells assuming a change in appearance. White blood cells decreased in the early part of the alarm stage, probably due to the inhibiting and destructive influence of the corticoids on lymphatic tissue formation. Today we know that immediately after a physical challenge our immune system is depressed for a period of time.

Third, he observed a degeneration in the gastrointestinal mucosa. We now know that if this condition continues, it results in gastrointestinal ulcers.

None of these alarm stage reactions were dangerous unless they persisted. They just showed that the organism was challenged. What Selye observed next was that when an organism was allowed to recover from a challenge, the organism adapted and developed more and better resources with which to meet future challenges.

ADAPTATION STAGE

In the alarm stage the organism experienced a drain on energy and resources, as well as some cellular destruction. No organism can maintain this stage continuously. It either has to resist the challenge or become exhausted and eventually die.

However, if the alarm stage is evoked repeatedly, intelligently, and consistently, allowing the organism to recover, the resource levels in the organism begin to rise (see Table 4.2). When this happens, the organism has entered the adaptation stage. In this stage, lasting up to 11 months, the energy and resources not only return to normal but are improved upon. Consequently, when the challenge occurs again, it will not seem as difficult. These gains in resources become noticeable, and performance and health improve.

Table 4.2

Structural	Oxygen Transport	Metabolic
Stronger Bones	Increased Heart Volume	Increased Aerobic Enzymes
Stronger Ligaments	Increased Heart Vascularization	Increased Anaerobic Enzymes
Stronger Tendons	Increased Heart Contractile Force	Increased Muscle ATP & PCr
Cartilage More Compressible	Increased Vagus Control	Increased Muscle RNA & DNA
Increased Muscle Protein	Increased Blood Volume	Increased Mitochondrial Protein
Decreased Neuron Inhibition	Increased Muscle Capillaries	Increased Glycogen Storage

Some Resources Improved by
Balancing Challenge and Recovery

Selye noted that the adaptation stage is influenced by the condition of the organism (for example, old versus young), the environment in which it finds itself (hot and humid versus cool), its previous conditioning to the specific challenge (trained versus untrained), and the level of challenge (intense versus moderate). Also, he observed that adaptation to one challenge will usually provide cross-resistance to other challenges.

Selye found that inducing the adaptation stage involves presenting the organism with repeated alarm stages followed by proper recovery so that the organism builds better resources with which to resist the challenge in the future. Adaptation is what occurs when people intelligently train themselves for athletic competition or use physical activity as a means to improve their health and well-being.

The next observation Selye made was that the adaptation stage did not last forever. The ability to adapt was limited. The closer an organism got to its potential, the harder it became to adapt. At some point challenges had to be removed so that the organism could experience a period of pure recovery. If this period was not made available to the organism, Selye's third stage, the exhaustion stage, appeared.

EXHAUSTION STAGE

The exhaustion stage is characterized by loss of the ability to adapt after prolonged exposure to a challenge or the addition of new challenges. Selye observed that when the challenge was drastically increased or prolonged over a long period of time or when new challenges were presented, any one of which might overload the system and deplete resources dangerously, the ability to adapt was lost.

In the adaptation stage, Selye observed anabolism, a building up of tissue. In the exhaustion stage, he observed symptoms similar to those of the first part of the alarm stage, but these symptoms persisted. Now there was catabolism, a tearing down of tissue and a reduction of resources.

In the exhaustion stage, not only will the individual's ability to adapt be lost, but unless the challenge is reduced or removed, the energy and resource level will continue to drop until it is below the original level. If relief is still not available, it will continue dropping through the nonspecific symptoms of illness that Selye observed, culminating in the appearance of a specific illness, an injury, or even death.

Several clues accompany the beginning of the exhaustion stage, clues that are easily observed, as shown in Table 4.2.

Table 4.3

Challenges Seem Harder
"Psyching up" Seems Harder
Irritated Easily
Disinterested in Surroundings
Abnormal Weight Loss
Poor Appetite
Poor Facial Skin Color and Texture
Fever Blisters/Canker Sores
Increased Muscle Soreness
Increased Joint Pain
Increased Exercise Heart Rate
Increased Morning Heart Rate

Symptoms of Exhaustion Stage

Interestingly enough, when these signs present themselves, athletes and/or the coach, if one is involved, often react by increasing challenges. They think that these signs mean that they are not working hard enough. In fact, though, Selye's theory predicts that the only workable solution is to reduce or remove the challenge. When a person enters too deeply into the exhaustion stage, probably after 7 to 10 days, the "season is over." There are not enough resources to resist and adapt to challenge, and illness or injury will ensue.

The exhaustion stage was to Selye a natural outcome because he felt that "even a fully inured organism cannot indefinitely maintain adaptation under continuous exposure to severe stress." He and others observed organisms so exhausted that neither the adrenal cortex nor the adrenal medulla could respond to a stimulus. He also observed that growth ceased and felt that it was because of the need to place all the body's resources at the disposal of functions that maintain homeostasis.

Following is a modified version of the graph Selye originally drew to depict his General Adaptation Syndrome.

Figure 4.1

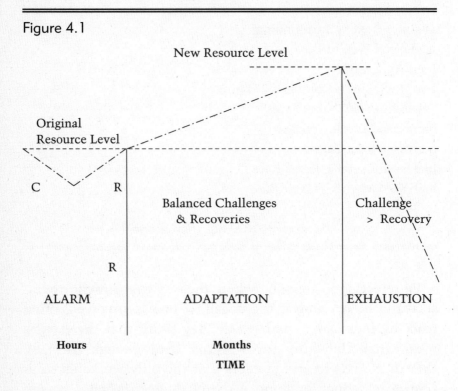

Modified Selye General Adaptation Syndrome

Modified Graph of Selye General Adapatation Syndrome
Alarm
> C = challenge (energy and resources needed to meet challenge)
>
> R = recovery (energy and resources return to original level)

Adaptation
> Repeated and balanced challenges and recoveries
>
> Energy and resource level improves, adapting to challenge

Exhaustion
> The sum of the challenges have exceeded the individual's ability to resist and adapt. The individual begins to lose energy and resources. The organic system needs relief!

Selye's theory explains why so many beginners burn out quickly. When people begin exercise programs, their uncertainty about what is right for them and their enthusiasm about beginning often prove to be a self-defeating combination. People become so enthusiastic that they overdo, falling almost immediately into Selye's exhaustion stage. Within a few weeks they become tired, bored, ill, or injured. They stop their physical activity and view themselves as failures.

If you respect the alarm stage by balancing challenge and recovery, adapt by intelligently repeating alarm stages, and listen to your body for clues to the exhaustion stage, you can enjoy a pleasant and productive association with physical activity for the rest of your life.

L.E.A.P. helps you do this because it is based upon understanding the need for balancing challenge and recovery. It provides you with a number that represents the amount of physical activity that is exactly right for you.

PART 2

THE 10-MINUTE L.E.A.P. PROGRAM

*I*n this section you will generate your two personal and special numbers: your Energy Conversion Number and your Energy Conversion Points. With these numbers you can define your physical self and set up a physical activity program that is right for you. You'll determine a place to start, a realistic goal at which to aim, and a very personal and flexible schedule to follow. You'll know the answers to the questions How often? How long? How hard?

CHAPTER 5

PHYSICAL CHARACTERISTICS AND LIFESTYLE CHOICES THAT AFFECT ENERGY CONVERSION

"Fate is often a choice."
—From *Triumph of the Human Spirit*, a video of the
1996 Paralympic Games

*H*ow do you know what type of physical activity is right for you? How do you know how often you should be physically active? How do you know how long you should be physically active? How do you know how intense the physical activity should be? Before these questions can be answered, you need to answer some questions about yourself. As you will see, different aspects of your life affect your ability to be physically active.

As an individual, your unique physical characteristics, lifestyle, and goals all merge to determine your ability to convert energy via physical activities at any particular moment in time.

The first question then becomes "How do I determine the amount of energy I have available to convert by being physically active?" The first thing a mentor would do in working with anyone who had a fitness goal—student, patient, adult, world-class athlete—would be to ask them questions about themselves.

L.E.A.P., like any good mentor, is no different. It will ask you to answer some questions in an autobiography. (The autobiography alone can be found in Appendix B.) Your auto-biography considers eight factors that affect your ability to convert energy, in order to determine your starting Energy Conversion Points (ECPs):

1. Age
2. Gender
3. Fat-free weight
4. Sleep
5. Relaxation
6. Nutrition
7. Current physical activity
8. Support and time

L.E.A.P. puts these factors together in a way that helps you determine your current VO2Max and translates that to your current ability to convert energy. Your personal VO2Max will be your main guideline in creating your own tailored L.E.A.P. program. It will also allow you to evaluate your health status or your position on the health continuum and to reevaluate your health as you change. The continuum can be represented as follows:

Figure 5.1

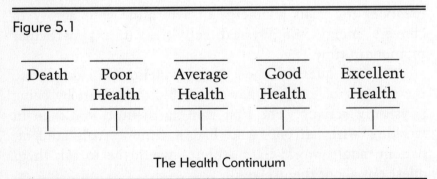

| Death | Poor Health | Average Health | Good Health | Excellent Health |

The Health Continuum

Health is a continuum, and you always reside somewhere on its sliding scale. Your position on the continuum is constantly changing and is usually under your control. A high VO2Max and the ability to convert energy efficiently are consistent with the upper end of the health continuum (good to excellent health).

Let's take a closer look at the eight factors that help make up your VO2Max—your ability to convert energy—one at a time.

AGE

"Most people live nowhere near their limits. They settle for an accelerated aging, an early and precipitous fall. They give aging a bad name. Too many people entering their forties are performing at physiological levels more appropriate to somebody sixty years old."

George Sheehan, cardiologist, author, runner

Why should we consider age when we are defining ability to convert energy? As we age it is obvious that no matter how well we eat, sleep, or exercise, time erodes our systems, leaving us functioning at a less efficient energy conversion level than the level we had in our youth. The decline in efficiency as we age is the result of evolution and "the thousand natural shocks that flesh is heir to." These factors are often aided and abetted by a lifestyle that does not give the care and maintenance of the body a high enough priority.

Evolution didn't prepare us well for life much over thirty. Not so long ago humans, if they were lucky, had fulfilled their biological purpose to reproduce by that age if they hadn't fallen prey to some nearby danger and died first. In terms of evolutionary time, that period was just a heartbeat ago. Although the body even then could live until seventy or eighty, it was definitely not the norm. Because this period is so recent from an evolutionary standpoint, the evolutionary mechanisms have had little chance to adapt to a longer life. As a result, when the body matures and stops growing, most cells in the body can no longer divide. They may be made up of constantly changing atoms, but they are no longer able to stay young by cell division. If we suffer an injury, the damaged cells aren't replaced by new cells; they are replaced by nonfunctioning scar tissue. Every time a cell is lost, a little bit of function is lost, and the remaining cells must pick up the slack. It is like a senescent free fall.

There is a theory that says cells can only divide a certain number of times. After the cell divides its predetermined number of times, division stops and the cell is no longer able to replace itself, eventually dying. After enough cells die, the organ dies, and then the organism. This programmed aging is determined by what is called the Hayflick number. Cells of different organs have different rates of division, but all, according to the theory, are ruled by their Hayflick number.

Cellular malfunction and death can also be provoked by disruptions to DNA, our genetic code. Ultraviolet radiation, gamma and X rays, and pollutants in our environment can cause damage to our DNA that results in abnormalities when protein structures are duplicated. Most of these genetic mutations are harmless, but cumulative genetic mutation results in proteins that are less stable and structures that are less functional. An enzyme (a protein key that unlocks chemical doors) that is less than fully functional could easily insert incorrect amino acids into a protein structure, changing the efficiency of the structure.

Accumulation of toxic waste is another environmental factor that affects cell efficiency and longevity by setting up mini waste dumps in cells. We also may suffer cumulative cell damage from free radicals, metabolic loose cannons that are a product of energy conversion. Our body, provided with proper nutrients and rest, can usually handle free radicals, but eventually they take a toll.

Some of the decline in cell efficiency is also due to the stress of just living. Because so much of modern life involves stressful situations, the role stress plays is increasingly significant. If we are constantly in Selye's alarm stage, catabolism, or breakdown of tissue, is dominant. Cortisol is made rather than testosterone, and cell function is directed away from cell maintenance and repair. Under constant alarm, the emotional center of the brain, the hippocampus, finds it difficult to turn off. It "overheats," destroying little bits of itself. Other research shows that excessive exposure to glucocorticoids, hormones released from the adrenal gland in response to stress, somehow blocks entry of glucose to the brain cells, denying them access to the only fuel they can use. Eventually even the ability to respond to stress can be lost. This upsets the ability to maintain homeostasis, further reducing the efficiency of the cells.

The result is that we age. Kidneys filter more slowly. Our immune system sometimes fails to recognize itself, resulting in autoimmune diseases, such as arthritis. Our vision and hearing slowly decline. Bone tissue decreases, making us more susceptible to broken bones. Cartilage tissue decreases, making us shorter. Muscle tissue decreases, reducing our strength. As a final insult, we can lose over one-half of our taste buds. Table 5.1 shows age-related declines between the ages of thirty, the approximate onset of aging in humans, and seventy-five, when death, on the average, interferes with aging.

Table 5.1

Structure/Function	% Decline
Brain Weight	8
Blood Supply to Brain	20
Nerve Conduction	10
Spinal Nerve Axons	37
Kidney Filtration	31
Bone Density	25
Muscle Mass	16
Muscle Strength	37
Lung Capacity	15
Maximum Heart Rate	25
Stroke Volume	30
Blood Volume	6
VO_2Max	44
Basal Metabolic Rate	12
Taste Buds	64
Body Fat	30% Increase

Age-Related Declines Between the Ages of 30 and 75

Can we stop aging? No. There are some factors that are beyond our control, such as the Hayflick number or our exposure to certain pollutants, either in the air we breathe or elsewhere. But we can control other factors to some extent, such as our reaction to stressful situations.

Can we slow aging down? Yes! There is much in aging that we can control. Much of accelerated aging is due to poor rest and nutritional habits and a lack of respect for the power of physical activity. The rate of aging is dependent upon the vigor of the organism. How quickly the effects of aging occur in your life can often be determined by you. You have the power to slow the aging process.

Brain cells can make new connections, even if a person is between the ages of sixty and ninety. Healthy, active older adults have scored improvements on intelligence tests. Learning and specific movements activate related areas of the brain, increasing activity and expanding connections in those areas. Learning also increases the strength of nerve transmissions and the quality of the nerve endings.

Decreases in bone density are associated with loss of calcium content. However, people with good dietary habits who incorporate physical activity in their lives don't usually experience as severe or as rapid a loss of calcium in their bones, because calcium uptake increases as physical activity increases. Studies of postmenopausal women on the same diet show that active women increase their calcium uptake while sedentary women lose calcium over the same period.

Wear and tear over time on connective tissues, such as cartilage, ligaments, and tendons, cause them to degenerate. This often results in compression of vertebrae, loss of flexibility, and arthritic conditions. The lungs, which are connective tissue, also lose elasticity, causing a reduction in breathing capacity. Those individuals who maintain an intelligent program of physical activity retain their height, are more limber, and work through arthritic conditions better than their sedentary contemporaries. Their vital capacity (the amount of air they can exchange) also remains nearly constant throughout their lives.

The amount of muscle protein decreases as we age. This contributes to a loss of muscle tone and strength. However, much of this loss can be attributed to lack of activity, to which muscle tissue is very responsive. The decrease in muscle protein in an unused muscle is rapid. A limb in a cast in a shortened position loses one-half its strength in the first 4 to 6 days. These losses are consistent with evolution because evolution does not maintain structures that are metabolically expensive but physiologically dormant.

However, muscle tissue is also very responsive to physical activity. It has been shown repeatedly that even if you start a strength building program in your seventies you can regain significant muscle function.

With age, the maximum heart rate decreases. The volume of the left ventricle, the chamber of the heart that pumps blood to all parts of the body except the lungs, also decreases. The lower maximum heart rate and the lower volume result in a decrease in the amount of blood the heart can pump per minute. Fit individuals, however, can raise their maximum heart rate higher than those who are not fit. Also, since the heart is a muscle and reacts like any other muscle when challenged with physical activity, the left ventricle in a fit person is stronger and more elastic. The result is that the blood volume pumped per beat need not decrease nearly as much as has been seen in sedentary individuals. The volume of blood the heart can pump per minute is a crucial component in VO_2Max.

As we get older, arteries, which contain connective tissue, experience a reduction in diameter and elasticity, raising blood pressure. The number of capillaries in the body is reduced, making each of the millions of cells a little farther from the blood supply. Physically fit people retain the elasticity of their arteries for a longer period of time, and the number of capillaries servicing cells can even be increased on a good aerobic program, ensuring a healthy blood supply to the cells.

VO_2Max declines about 10% per decade after age twenty-five. A consistent physical activity program can slow the decline so significantly that a physically active seventy-five-year-old can have a better VO_2Max than an inactive forty-five-year-old. The following table compares the VO_2Max changes for two people who both had a VO_2Max of 50.0 at age twenty-five (see Table 5.2).

Table 5.2

Age	VO2Max Inactive	VO2 Max Active
25	50.0	50.0
35	45.0	48.0
45	<u>40.5</u>	46.1
55	36.5	44.2
65	32.8	42.5
75	29.5	<u>40.8</u>

Age-Related VO2Max Comparisons

Another indication that aging need not be uniformly detrimental to the oxygen consumption systems is that the highest ranked female 1500-meter runner in the world in 1994 was forty-four years old!

The fact that the ability to convert energy slows as we age cannot be completely laid at the feet of the aging process. Some of this decline is due to changes in body composition. In many cases our individual body weight increases due to an increase in fat tissue. With the change in the fat-free-weight–to–fat weight ratio, even if our weight stays the same, our body composition does not. Since muscle tissue converts energy about nine times faster than fat tissue, the metabolic rate is reduced. Physically active people do not lose their ability to convert energy as they age as rapidly as their sedentary counterparts, because their fat-free-weight–to–fat weight ratio stays higher.

It was once thought that sexual decline with age was unavoidable. It was then found that the decline was as closely related to inactivity and poor diet as to age. Physically unfit men over sixty tend to have up to six times the sexual problems as those who are fit. For men over seventy, the difference is forty times.

Active people can enjoy satisfying sex almost to the end of their lives. Results of interviews with over 800 healthy, active men and women between sixty and ninety-one revealed that most continued to be very interested in sex and enjoyed it as much as or more than when they were younger. Older women required more foreplay to attain wetness, but older men could delay ejaculation longer. This combination can produce very enjoyable sexual experiences. As Dr. Paul Fleming is quoted as saying "Older people can't have sex three times an hour, but they are better equipped to do it once and make it last an hour."

The effects of aging needn't occur as fast as they do in contemporary society. Physically active people can be 10 to 30 years younger in structure and function than their sedentary contemporaries, as shown in Table 5.3.

Table 5.3

System	Function	% Decline Sedentary	% Decline Active
Skeletal	Bone Density	25	9
Muscular	Strength	37	13
	Mass	16	6
Cardiovascular	Maximum Heart Rate	25	9
	Blood Volume	6	2
	VO2Max	44	15
Respiratory	Lung Capacity	15	5
Overall Body	Ability to Convert Calories	12	5
	Body Fat	30% Increase	13% Increase

Comparison of the Effects of Aging between the Ages of 30 and 75 in Sedentary and Physically Active People

Being physically active is simply doing what nature intended. When you obey the Law of Conservation of Energy, pay your respects to entropy, and apply force to overcome inertia, you can dramatically delay aging.

However, you can't stop getting chronologically older and the inevitable decline, no matter how much you have slowed it down. Therefore, in the L.E.A.P. autobiography, you need to use your correct age. Other lifestyle factors in the autobiography modify the effects of your age score. Depending on the answers, you will see that they potentiate aging or delay aging, decreasing or increasing your ability to convert energy.

GENDER

Gender is the second major factor in your personal profile. There are physiological differences between the sexes that result in different performance levels. As late as the 1956 Olympics it was thought that women could not perform as strenuously as men. A women's 800-meter race was held in the 1928 Olympics, but viewing the effort expended by the women runners so upset officials that women were not allowed to run anything longer than the 200 meters until the 1960 Rome Olympics, when the 800-meter race was reinstated.

In fact, gender differences are not as great as previously thought. The women's record for the 10,000-meter run is now better than the men's 1948 Olympic record of the great Emil Zatopek. Many women running today have times in the marathon that would have enabled them to win every men's Olympic marathon through 1956.

A major factor in closing the gap is that social stigmas that once discouraged women from training effectively have evaporated. The differences continue to lessen as women train more. But despite the closing gap, there are still differences. One of those differences is body fat. In 1980 Cureton and Sparling, two well-respected exercise physiologists, wrote in a research report that "Since sex-specific, essential fat cannot be eliminated by diet or training, it provides part of a biological justification for . . . different . . . expectations for men and women." Why do women generally have more body fat than men?

Before going through puberty, male and female performance is about the same. It is not unusual for a girl to beat a boy in anything. After puberty the major difference seems to be testosterone. Before puberty both males and females have concentrations of testosterone in blood plasma of about 40 ng/dl (.00000001431 ounces per quart). After puberty females maintain about the same concentration of testosterone and also secrete the hormone estrogen. Males, however, have normal plasma testosterone concentrations of 600 ng/dl (.0000002147 ounces per quart), or fifteen times as much testosterone.

Since testosterone increases muscle tissue, retards accumulation of fat, and increases hemoglobin content, the work capacity of the male increases. Estrogen, on the other hand, increases the accumulation of adipose tissue and retards the development of muscle tissue. The testosterone differences, which result in physiological and anatomical differences, give males an advantage in physical performance. Having a greater muscle mass and less fat results in a strength-to-weight ratio difference that favors men by about 15%.

In addition, because of the testosterone difference men tend to have broader shoulders, upon which to build more upper body strength, and a larger chest cavity, which gives them a greater lung volume. Men also tend to have greater bone density and therefore to be less subject to overuse injuries affecting the bones. Women, on the other hand, tend to have wider hips, causing a difference in the angle the lower extremities make with the hips. Biomechanically this makes it harder for women to sprint as fast. But it also gives women a lower center of gravity, which results in better balance. Men tend to have a higher volume of blood and a greater concentration of red blood cells, resulting in more hemoglobin, the oxygen carrying component of the red blood cells. The volume of the heart tends to be greater in males, as well as the muscle mass of the heart. This means that the male heart tends to pump more blood per beat, while the female heart must beat faster to pump an equal amount of blood.

Another physiological factor that contributes to differences in gender performance is that women, up to a certain age, have the additional genetic requirement to menstruate. The blood lost through menstruation causes iron loss. The iron loss, combined with lower rates of iron absorption and often lower iron intake, can result in anemia, which further decreases the ability to carry oxygen. Also, during the premenstrual phase of the cycle, 1 to 2 kg of fluid are retained, making physical activity more difficult.

Many women can perform better than many men in athletic and fitness events. But the best men, due to testosterone-based physiological differences, will outperform the best women in any specific event. The physiological differences in body fat, muscle mass, lung capacity, blood volume, hemoglobin content, and cardiac output result in the male's higher VO2Max. These facts are considered in the L.E.A.P. autobiography when determining your VO2Max and are numerically accounted for in the Modified Body Mass Index formula in the fat-free weight portion of the autobiography.

FAT-FREE WEIGHT

The third factor L.E.A.P. considers in determining your unique fitness profile is body composition because body weight, or mass, is important in the conversion of energy. If you think about it, it's obvious. Carrying a heavy trunk takes more effort than toting around a small briefcase. To bring science into the picture, you may recall that energy conversion is required to move a mass through a distance or against gravity. The amount of energy you convert is determined by the formula

Energy (joules) = kg x m^2/sec^2

For example, if two people who were equal in all respects, except that one weighed 65 kg (143 pounds) and the other 88 kg (193 pounds), ran 1500 meters in 8 minutes, the first would have to convert about 151 calories and the second about 205 calories.

Joules of Energy$_{Person\ 1}$ = 65 kg x $(1500\ m)^2/(480\ sec)^2$
= 635 joules
Calories = 635 joules/4.2 joules /cal = 151 calories
Joules of Energy$_{Person\ 2}$ = 88 kg x $(1500\ m)^2/(480\ sec)^2$
= 860 joules
Calories = 860 joules /4.2 joules /cal = 205 calories

But it turns out that when it comes to the human body, all weight is not the same. More important than the total mass, or weight, in everyday life, is the composition of that weight. The type of weight you have determines how efficient you are in converting energy.

There are two basic components of body composition: fat-free weight and fat weight. Fat-free weight is made up of bone, blood, organs, and muscle. Fat weight is made up of essential and nonessential fat. These tissues influence your basal metabolic rate, the rate at which you convert energy to sustain life. They also influence your metabolism throughout the day and when you are physically active.

Fat-free tissue is much more active than fat tissue, converting about nine times as many calories per day as fat tissue. Fat-free tissue may convert about 39.6 cal/kg/day, while fat tissue may convert 4.4 cal/kg/day. Table 5.4 shows an example of two people who weigh 65 kg (143 pounds) but have different body compositions.

Table 5.4

	Lean Person	Not Lean Person
Total Body Weight (kg)	65	65
% Fat-Free Weight	82.5	70
% Fat Weight	17.5	30
Fat-Free Kilograms	53.6	45.5
Fat Kilograms	11.4	19.5
Calories Converted/Day by Fat-Free Weight	2123	1802
Calories Converted/Day by Fat Weight	50	86
Total Calories Converted/Day	2173	1888

Caloric Expenditure of Two People Who Weigh the Same but Have Different Body Composition

The difference between the calories converted each day is 285. Since 1 pound of fat is equivalent to about 3500 calories, the person whose body composition contains only 17.5% fat converts enough calories to consume an extra pound of fat every 12 days. This person will also lose fat weight more easily, not gain it as readily, and will be able to enjoy more food. L.E.A.P. will help you begin to shift the fat-free weight–to–fat weight ratio in the right direction.

It also turns out that your height and your frame, which are dependent upon bone, and your muscle bulk, which is dependent upon muscle tissue, are fat-free tissues that affect the rate at which you consume calories. For example, the taller you are, the higher your metabolism. The difference in metabolism between someone 5'8" and someone 5'10" may be 70 calories per day or about 35 calories per inch per day. L.E.A.P. considers these factors in determining your VO2Max.

Though you can have tests done in a lab to learn your body composition, there's a fairly accurate way for you to estimate it. L.E.A.P. uses this technique in showing you how to determine your VO2Max.

SLEEP

For truly lasting and potent fitness gains, regular and good recovery habits are essential. Recovery is giving your body the time and the right conditions to recover from challenge. This means you need to remove challenges for a period of time and place yourself in a situation where the body can focus on recovery.

Sleep is a major component of recovery, which is why sleep is a part of your autobiography. Of all the biological components of adaptation, sleep is probably the least well understood. But it does seem clear that sleep has restoration of the body as a major goal and that sleep is an integral part of our biological rhythm. Biological, or circadian, rhythms are governed by an internal clock and extend back further than human life. These rhythms can be found in the plant and animal kingdom and in one-celled organisms and are still with us today because of their obvious survival value. A period of inactivity allows dangers to be avoided and resources to be conserved. At the beginning of human evolution, active pursuits were limited by darkness, which at the same time increased danger and risks. It made biological sense to not only find a place to protect oneself but also conserve energy during the night.

As more research is produced it becomes apparent that whatever the reasons, sleep is vital for normal function. This period of relative inactivity is a time when cells are renewed and healed, a time when all the concentration of the body can focus on rebuilding. It is known that hormones that enhance the synthesis of red blood cells and bone are released when we sleep and that poor sleep habits decrease performance. Serious sleep deprivation can cause mental disturbances.

What can you do to maximize your sleep recovery time? First, don't take in any caffeine or alcohol within 3 hours of going to bed. Caffeine is a stimulant and will make it more difficult to get to sleep. Likewise, alcohol is a substance that has to be neutralized by the body. This is done in the liver, which also is important in the rebuilding process. When it must detoxify alcohol, it can't efficiently complete the process of renewal. Alcohol taken within several hours of going to sleep also interferes with the stages of sleep.

Better sleep occurs when it has a regular place in the 24-hour cycle. Try to get to bed about the same time each night. Each of us has an internal clock that works best on a regular schedule. Establish a pattern that enhances the efficiency of your body clock. Try to avoid sleeping longer on weekends because that will disturb the rhythm. This will not disturb sleep as much as shift work, but nevertheless, light and activity patterns occurring at different times of the day than usual send messages to the body that disturb circadian rhythms. Getting up at the same time, even if you got to bed later, will help you maintain, or reset, your body clock. It may also encourage you to get to sleep at approximately the same time each night. It turns out that regular physical activity can also help reset your body clock.

I recommend sleeping in a quiet, dark room with fresh, cool air on a firm mattress to provide the most satisfactory sleep environment. Sleeping on a wool mattress cover in a semifetal position also seems to enhance sleep.

Having a bedtime routine and relaxing before you sleep can help you get to sleep sooner and sleep better. Little things like brushing your teeth, tightening and relaxing muscles for a minute or so after lying down, or reading can tell your body, "This is what I do before I go to sleep, so get ready." A routine, especially reading, also helps take your mind off current or future stressful situations.

Maintaining a rhythm helps you wake up on your own. It is better for you to wake up naturally and lie quietly in bed a few minutes than to be jolted awake by an alarm.

RELAXATION

For many reasons pressure has become the name of the game in 20th century living. This problem is only compounded by the fact that many individuals in industrial nations have trouble understanding the value of rest, relaxation, and relief from pressure. As a result, it has been estimated that significantly more than half of all visits to health care professionals are due to pressure- or stress-related causes. This is why lab tests reveal organic causes less than one-quarter of the time. Even when lab tests reveal organic problems, stress can have played a contributory role.

Stress is the response of the body to challenge, and challenges need not always be unpleasant. For example, winning the lottery might be pleasant, but I guarantee your body would react to it as to a challenge. The key is how much control we exert over our stressors. We must control them, not have them control us.

If challenge is perceived as a commitment we voluntarily accept, are interested in meeting, and feel we have some control over, we react with action and involvement. This is a healthy acceptance of the challenge, and our heightened resources go toward constructively meeting the challenge. Action gives the biochemical cascade of responses to stress a place to go.

If we perceive the challenge as a threat, feel helpless, and are filled with anxiety instead of anticipation, we become "stressed out." Repeated or prolonged exposure to such stressors, especially negative everyday minor stressors, results in physical and emotional exhaustion. The results of stress have been seen in all the systems of the body, including the brain, where bombardment with stress hormones destroys hormone receptor sites.

When we perceive a threat, as we learned in the chapter on Selye, our body prepares us to meet the threat. Smooth muscle in the digestive tract relaxes, reducing the energy requirement for the digestive system. Blood vessels in the respiratory system open wider, increasing blood flow to respiratory muscles and to the capillaries in the alveoli. The diaphragm pushes down, enlarging the chest cavity so that more oxygen can be made available to the alveoli. The heart rate increases and the heart muscle expands and beats more powerfully so that more blood is pumped per beat. Vessels in the intestines and skin constrict, while vessels in the skeletal muscles open. This increases the delivery of blood carrying valuable oxygen and energy sources to the skeletal muscles. Liver glycogen is changed to glucose, while fatty acids are released from fat cells. Both of these energy sources are delivered to the muscle cells by the blood. Nervous system sensitivity is increased, enhancing reaction time. The body is ready to use these resources to do something special.

In modern industrial society, this reaction is often stimulated by frustration or anger, which is a perceived or emotional threat instead of a physical one. What happens? The body idles in neutral much too fast, blood pressure builds, resources are wasted. Much like a car, the body loses its tuning and parts begin to degenerate. No outlet for the "fight or flight" response contributes to the development of degenerative diseases.

Why does the body seem to fight itself and cause bad things to happen to itself when faced with a perception of a threat? In the past, these threats were real. As a result, the risk of this type of wear and tear on the body was relatively less severe. But the legacy continues today and probably not for the best. As Dr. Herbert Benson points out in his book *Timeless Healing*, this reaction is now hardwired into our bodies.

We inherited from earlier generations the physiologic ability to fight effectively or to run away from danger because our ancestors were unlikely to survive without it. We retained a genetic wisdom of the ages, designed to secure our future on earth.

Evolution couldn't keep up with the pace of change in industrial society. It couldn't account for the fact that today we may perceive something as a threat that is not really life-threatening. Most stressors today are false alarms, but as Dr. Benson adds, "'fight or flight' is a knee-jerk reaction that has been ingrained for millions of years." Perception of a threat, such as irritations caused by being stuck in traffic, an argument with a fellow worker, or a deadline, triggers the reaction but does not allow a physical response. Your body is prepared for a physical response, but in our society a physical response is not acceptable. After all, your life is not threatened. Or is it? What happens if constant stimulation of the "fight or flight" response occurs with no place for it to go?

The body becomes exhausted and begins to break down. Almost every condition we go to physicians for can have roots in the calling forth of the "fight or flight" response. Cardiovascular problems, immune problems, psychological problems, metabolic problems—all can be related to a prolonged, frequent, unrequited elicitation of "fight or flight." Constant tension, with little relief, affects your ability to convert energy. Physical activity provides a positive outlet for these "turned on" resources. It dissipates the energy, returning the body to equilibrium. Physical activity gives stress a healthy place to go.

Like the other questions in the autobiography, the questions about relaxation were selected from a wide range of choices, and they correlate well with your ability to relax. That ability has major implications for the efficiency with which you convert energy and use resources.

In Appendix G you can find a short description of how to elicit the "relaxation response." This technique was developed by Dr. Benson to help you to live healthfully with the stressors in your life.

NUTRITION

The next factor L.E.A.P. considers in your autobiography is your nutritional status. Food is your source of energy, your link to the sun. In balancing challenge and recovery you must start with nutrition. If you do not provide the body with the raw material to rebuild structures and restore energy, no recovery or future development can take place.

The L.E.A.P. questions do not ask about how much of this or how many servings of that you consume. Instead L.E.A.P. looks at your nutritional attitudes, which reflect your diet and how well you eat. L.E.A.P. asks about food groups because by eating from all the groups you ensure that your body will get all the nutrients. While most foods have a variety of nutrients, some food groups are better at supplying certain nutrients. Meats and legumes (beans and seeds) supply amino acids. Grains usually have high levels of carbohydrates. Vegetables and fruits contain a broad spectrum of vitamins and minerals and provide fiber. Dairy products are rich in amino acids, minerals, and fats. Getting a balanced diet means getting enough protein, carbohydrate, fat, minerals, vitamins, and fiber. The best way to do this is to eat from all food groups.

L.E.A.P. asks whether you read labels. If you pick up food just because it tastes good and don't care what the ingredients are, this suggests you could probably eat better and con-vert energy more efficiently than you are doing now.

Like reading labels, eating organically grown foods also suggests several things about the health of your diet. Even though much that is added to food is not dangerous, your body must still use resources to deal with any substances added to your food that your body is not going to use. Once colors, flavors, binders, preservatives, pesticides, and insecti-cides enter the body, they do not magically disappear. Resources must be committed to eliminate or store them. It's better if they do not enter the body in the first place.

Purchasing and preparing food as close to fresh as possi-ble is a fourth factor that reflects your nutritional health. The further you get from fresh organic food, the more nutri-ents are lost and the more nutrient-free or detrimental sub-stances are added. Fast food, the ubiquitous hamburgers and fries, and junk food, like doughnuts and chips, are examples of foods that are many steps removed from fresh.

Now I'm going to attack an institution, coffee. I know people "need" their caffeine, but caffeine potentiates the body's "fight or flight" response. In addition to that, caffeine is something that your body gets used to. The more you drink, the less the kick, and then the more you have to drink. If used sparingly it can help you through challenges, but if taken three, four, or five times a day it will soon become just another habit that does little that is good for your body.

Excessive use of alcohol and smoking also negatively affect your ability to convert energy.

I am not trying to take away the joy of eating. I like food as well as anyone else and I enjoy what I eat. I like junk food, especially chocolate. But I have learned that you can enjoy eat-ing good foods and not totally deprive yourself of the foods that just seem to taste good (those that are salty, fatty, or sweet). For 25 years my daughter and I have more or less followed what we informally call "The Big Day Diet." All that means is that for 6 days of the week we try to eat intelligently, a little junk food allowed, and on the 7th we eat whatever we want and as much as we want. If you're interested, you can find this diet described in more detail in Appendix F. Once you've read those pages, you will probably have 95% of all the eating information you'll ever need. If you can eat the "Big Day" way for the rest of your life, you will never have to worry about nutrition again, and you'll enjoy it.

CURRENT PHYSICAL ACTIVITY

Of course, L.E.A.P. takes your present level of physical activity into account in creating your profile. Your current activity pattern may or may not be what is best for you at this time, but it does help to evaluate your current ability to convert energy.

L.E.A.P. asks you about your activity category. It also asks how often, how long, and how intense your current physical activities are. Your activity category indicates what your goals are likely to be. It can be assumed that someone who is currently inactive will have different aspirations than someone who is competing in age-group competitions. Your activity level also probably indicates not only your current level of fitness but how firm your commitment is to physical activity.

Frequency and duration estimate the time factor and indicate how many minutes per week you are currently devoting to physical activity. Intensity estimates what %VO2Max you use when you are active. Intensity in both directions—too much or too little—has a major impact on your energy conversion due to the level of response it elicits from the body's "fight or flight" mechanisms.

Your level of current activity also addresses the issue of basal metabolism. If you are currently active, you have a higher percentage of muscle tissue than if you are sedentary. As the amount of muscle tissue increases, your metabolism increases because muscle tissue is metabolically more active than fat tissue. In addition, after you work out, your metabolism does not return to preexercise levels for 1 to 2 hours.

SUPPORT AND TIME

L.E.A.P. recognizes that support and time influence your ability to sustain physical activity. If your partner, family, friends, or employer understand that physical activity will help you, and therefore ultimately help them, it will be easier for you to maintain a fitness program. If, on the other hand, you hear comments like "Are you going to work out again?" or "I don't want you to work out during company time," being physically active is going to be much harder.

If your partner or friends share your activity, you get a major boost in your ability to make physical activity a part of your life. If you have workout partners, you are more likely to remain active because you tend to reinforce each other on those days you feel you are too busy to work out or just don't feel like it. It's surprising how often you come away from those workouts feeling less tired and being more effective than you were before.

There are things you can do to develop support. A polite but frank explanation of the benefits to you and to your family, friends, and employer is a place to start. You can also use some physical effort around your home to do your share of the chores. I used to hate to rake leaves until I realized that not only did it make my partner feel good that I was contributing to the upkeep of our home, but it also contributed to converting energy just like any other physical activity. So what if it wasn't running or playing a game? It converted calories, it was an investment in all my future activity via ongoing support, and it helped our relationship.

Even in situations where employers have no wellness programs, with a little imagination and determination you can be active. For 6 years I taught in a high school. I had five classes, a study hall, and one free period each day. I also had lunch duty on certain days and coached for almost 3 hours after school every day. No one in the school administration said they would like me to work out. Yet every day I had completed a 5-mile run before 1:30 P.M. And I didn't do it in the early morning. I am not an early morning workout person.

What I did was make a deal with the school administration and the two other teachers in my department. I would take all the general biology classes. These were classes the other science teachers didn't like to teach. In return I was given my free period just before lunch and my study hall just after lunch. I got permission to give my lunch duty "free lunch ticket" to a teacher who said he would do my lunch duty for the free lunch. I also asked to teach one class in the physiology of exercise to the college-bound high school students. It worked out great. The other science teachers were happy. Jim got his free lunch. The administration was happy because the staff was happier. And I got to run 5 miles in the middle of each school day. I know I was a healthier person. And I know I was a much better teacher in the afternoon than I would have been without the exercise. An added bonus—the general biology students turned out to be great kids when you got to know them.

I not only got support, but I fit it into a very time-sensitive day. Not taking the time to be active by using the excuse that you can't afford the time is not acceptable. The truth for your body is that you can't afford not to make time available to be physically active.

In Dr. James Rippe's book, *Fit for Success*, Richard Snyder, CEO of a major publishing company, is quoted as saying, "I make my time for physical activity as important as any other appointment on my calendar." I can't tell you how many times that thought has made me drop something to do a workout that I might not otherwise have taken the time to do.

A few years ago I had a small office in Eugene with a few employees. This time I was the employer and didn't have to ask permission to be active. But we were very busy, and throughout the day I was constantly on the phone. It turned out that the local YMCA had basketball open gym between 2 and 4 P.M. every Monday, Wednesday, and Friday. I love to play basketball, so I decided to schedule my workouts during that time on those days. One employee was very concerned because, as she said, "The phone will ring off the hook for you during that time." I said to tell them what I was doing; they would appreciate it and get used to calling at other times. They did get used to it, and I got some of the most enjoyable workouts I've ever had. The point is, if you really value physical activity and are not just giving it lip service, you can explore your situation and figure out how to make your "time for physical activity as important as any other appointment on your calendar."

By taking account of all these factors: age, gender, fat-free weight, sleep patterns, relaxation ability, nutritional habits, current physical activity level, support and time, L.E.A.P. generates an amazingly accurate picture of your current ability to convert energy. Now its time to plunge into the autobiography and find how well you consume oxygen and convert energy.

CHAPTER 6

THE AUTOBIOGRAPHY

*T*his chapter is a workbook for you. Please write in it so that you have all the answers you need to determine your VO2Max and your starting Energy Conversion Points (ECPs). Appendix B is a short form of the autobiography you can use to reevaluate your VO2Max as aspects of your life change.

Table 6.1

Age	Score
30 or less	4
31 to 40	3
41 to 65	2
Over 65	1

AGE SCORE = _____

Example*:

	Marlene		Dick	
Age	=	>41	Age	=	59
Age Score	=	2	Age Score	=	2

Age

*For the examples throughout this autobiography section, I will use Marlene, whom you met in Chapter 3, and myself. I believe that a coach or mentor should always be willing to do anything he or she asks the athlete or the person seeking information to do. The night before the 1500-meter final in the 1960 Rome Olympics, Percy Cerutty, who was coaching world record holder and eventual Gold Medal winner Herb Elliott, asked Herb to come to a practice track. There Cerutty, who was over sixty at the time, ran a mile in around 6 minutes. He said, "Herb, you will run faster, but you won't run harder."

GENDER

The gender adjustment is accounted for in the fat-free-weight segment you will do next.

During pregnancy there are additional energy costs that must be considered. These are the energy needs of the fetus, the increased metabolic rate, and the additional weight to be carried about. Exercise is beneficial during pregnancy and should be done, but it should be modified to account for the additional requirement.

Enter –1 if pregnant. Enter 0 if not.

Pregnancy Score _____

FAT-FREE WEIGHT

It takes several steps to estimate your fat-free weight, but you will find that it is a very valuable number.

Step 1. Frame, Leanness, Muscle Bulk/Tone Adjustment

Use the Body Composition Adjustment table to estimate as honestly as you can your frame size, leanness, and muscle bulk/tone.

Frame size estimates the amount of bone that contributes to your body weight. To get a quick estimate of your frame size, take your dominant hand and wrap the thumb and middle finger around the wrist of your other hand behind the bony prominence. If the thumb and finger touch, your frame size is average. If they don't touch, it is large or very large. It they overlap, it is small or very small.

Your leanness score estimates the amount of fat you have at this time.

Muscle bulk/tone estimates the amount of muscle tissue you have at this time.

Choose one answer in each of the categories and add the three scores together.

Table 6.2

Frame	Frame Score	Leanness	Leanness Score	Muscle Bulk	Muscle Score
Very Small	–2	Overweight or Too Lean	–4	It's There Somewhere	–3
			-3		–2
Small	–1	Not Lean	–2	Less Than Other People	–1
Average	0	Average	0	Average	0
Large	+1	Lean	+2	More Than Other People	+2
			+3		+3
Very Large	+2	Very Lean	+4	Much More Than Other People	+4
Your Score ____			____		____
			ADJUSTMENT SCORE		____

Body Composition Adjustment

Now take your adjustment score and add it to 21 if it is a plus number or subtract it from 21 if it is a minus number.

21+ or – Adjustment = _____

This number is your Frame, Leanness, Muscle Bulk/Tone Adjustment.

Example:

	Marlene	
Frame	= Average	= 0
Leanness	= Lean	= +2
Muscle Bulk/Tone	= Average	= 0
Adjustment Score	= +2	

Frame, Leanness, Muscle Bulk Adjustment = 21 + 2 = 23

	Dick	
Frame	= Average	= 0
Leanness	= Lean	= +2
Muscle Bulk/Tone	= Above Average	= +2
	Total Score	= +4

Frame, Leanness, Muscle Bulk Adjustment = 21 + 4 = 25

Step 2. L.E.A.P. Modified Body Mass Index

The Body Mass Index, which compares your weight with your height, is modified from metric to English units and for gender. It is used as a general estimate of body composition, which is then more accurately fine-tuned by the Frame, Leanness, Muscle Bulk/Tone Adjustment you just completed.

Divide your body weight in pounds by your height in inches squared. Then, if you are male, multiply that by 1130; if you are female, multiply by 1270. Round off to one decimal place. This is your Modified Body Mass Index.

$$\frac{Body\ Weight\ (pounds)\ x\ 1130\ (males)\ or\ 1270(females)}{Height\ (inches)\ x\ Height\ (inches)}$$

EQUATION

Males
____ *(pounds)* x *1130* ÷ ____ *(inches)* x ____ *(inches)*= ____ *(to one decimal place)*

Females
____ *(pounds) x 1270 ÷ ____ (inches) x ____ (inches)=* ____
(to one decimal place)

Your Modified Body Mass Index =____

Example:

Marlene
Body Weight = 143 Pounds
Height = 67 inches
Modified Body Mass Index = 143 x 1270 ÷ 4489 = 40.5

Dick
Body Weight = 194 Pounds
Height = 75 inches
Modified Body Mass Index = 194 x 1130 ÷ 5625 = 39.0

Step 3. Estimated % Fat Weight

Subtract the Frame, Leanness, Muscle Bulk/Tone Adjustment from the Modified Body Mass Index. This is an estimate of the percentage of fat weight in your body.

Estimated % Fat Weight = Body Mass Index – Frame, Leanness, Muscle Bulk Adjustment

_____ – _____ = _____

Your Estimated % Fat Weight = _____

Example:

Marlene
Body Mass Index = 40.5
Frame, Leanness, Muscle Bulk/
Tone Adjustment = 23
Estimated % Fat Weight = 40.5 – 23 = 17.5

Dick

Body Mass Index	=	39.0
Frame, Leanness, Muscle Bulk/ Tone Adjustment	=	25
Estimated % Fat Weight	=	39.0 – 25 = 14.0

Step 4. Estimated % Fat-Free Weight

Now, instead of thinking of fat weight, get in the habit of thinking of fat-free weight. To get your percentage of fat-free weight, subtract your estimated percentage of fat weight from 100.

Estimated % Fat-Free Weight = 100 – Estimated % Fat Weight

100 – _____ = _____

Your Estimated % Fat-Free Weight = _____

Example:

Marlene

Estimated % Fat Free Weight   =   100 – 17.5 = 82.5

Dick

Estimated % Fat Free Weight   =   100 – 14.0 = 86.0

Table 6.3 provides general guidelines for various levels of fat-free weight. Age will make some difference in this rating but can be ignored for our purposes because the percentages listed are generally within the categories for all age groups. If you are an athlete competing at a high level and find yourself in the Usually Too High category, you can use 3 as your score instead of 2.5. The reason the score is lower is because at this level of fat-free weight you are very close to being too lean.

Table 6.3

Level of Fat-Free Weight	% Men	% Women	Fat-Free Weight Score
Usually Too High	≥92	≥88	2.5
Very Healthy	≥86<92	≥82<88	4
Healthy	≥77<86	≥73<82	3
Could Be Higher	≥70<77	≥66<73	2
Too Low	<70	<66	1

Fat-Free Weight Score

Your Fat-Free Weight Score = _____

Example:

Marlene

Estimated % Fat Free Weight = 82.5

Fat-Free Weight Score = 4

Dick

Estimated % Fat Free Weight = 86.0

Fat-Free Weight Score = 4

If you want to get an idea of how your weight is distributed, multiply your body weight by the percentages. When you weigh yourself it should be done in the same state of dress or undress and at the same time each day. I ask my athletes to weigh themselves in the morning, nude, just after they get up, after they void and before they eat.

Body Weight = _____

Fat Weight = Body Weight x Estimated % Fat Weight ÷ 100

= _____

_____ × _____ ÷100 = _____

Fat-Free Weight = Body Weight x Estimated % Fat-Free Weight ÷ 100 = _____

_____ × _____ ÷100 = _____

Example:

Marlene

Body Weight = 143

Estimated % Fat Weight = 17.5%

Fat Weight = 143 × .175 = 25 pounds

Estimated % Fat Free Weight = 82.5%

Fat-Free Weight = 143 × .825 = 118 pounds

Dick

Body Weight = 194

Estimated % Fat Weight = 14.0%

Fat Weight = 194 × .140 = 27 pounds

Estimated % Fat Free Weight = 86.0%

Fat-Free Weight = 194 × .860 = 167 pounds

Up to a point, the idea is to try to increase the fat-free weight in the body. You will notice that when the percentage of fat-free weight is too high, the fat-free weight score is reduced because there is a danger of exhausting the fat resources that the body requires.

Additionally, just losing weight is not the answer. If you crash diet or if you do not combine good eating habits with intelligent activity, you stand a good chance of losing too much muscle tissue, the most metabolically active tissue in the body. Losing muscle tissue lowers metabolism and does not improve health and fitness

SLEEP

Table 6.4

Question	Usually	Sometimes	Not Usually	Score
Do you drink beverages with caffeine or alcohol within 3 hours of going to bed?	1	2	3	_____
Do you have a relaxing routine before going to bed?	3	2	1	_____
Do you go to bed about the same time each night?	4	2	1	_____
Is there fresh air in your bedroom?	3	2	1	_____
Is your bedroom dark and quiet?	3	2	1	_____
Is your sleeping surface too hard/too soft?	1	2	3	_____
Do you have trouble getting to sleep?	1	2	4	_____
If you wake up during the night, do you have trouble getting back to sleep?	1	2	3	_____
Do you get up about the same time, even on weekends?	4	2	1	_____
Do you get up naturally, without an alarm?	3	2	1	_____
Are you still tired when you get up?	1	2	3	_____
Do you get the amount of sleep you feel you need?	4	2	0	_____
			Total	_____
		Total ÷ 12		_____

Sleep Score

In the Sleep segment, round off to two decimal places.

Your Sleep Score = _____

In areas where improvements in lifestyle can influence your ability to convert energy, I'll give you a grade, and you can go back and look at some of those lifestyle patterns or living habits you might want to modify to improve your grade. When your grade improves, your VO2Max improves, and your ability to convert energy improves with it.

Table 6.5

Sleep Grade	Range
A	2.93 – 3.33
B	2.43 – 2.92
C	1.59 – 2.42
D	1.09 – 1.58
F	0.83 – 1.08

Example:

		Marlene		
Caffeine/alcohol	=	Not Usually	=	3
Relaxing routine	=	Sometimes	=	2
Same time to bed	=	Sometimes	=	2
Fresh air	=	Usually	=	3
Dark/quiet	=	Usually	=	3
Too hard/too soft	=	Not Usually	=	3
Getting to sleep	=	Sometimes	=	2
Back to sleep	=	Sometimes	=	2
Up at same time	=	Sometimes	=	2
Up naturally	=	Sometimes	=	2
Still tired	=	Sometimes	=	2
Sleep you need	=	Sometimes	=	2
		Total	=	28
Total ÷ 12	=	Sleep Score	=	2.33
		Grade	=	C

Dick

Caffeine/alcohol	=	Not Usually	=	3
Relaxing routine	=	Usually	=	3
Same time to bed	=	Usually	=	4
Fresh air	=	Usually	=	3
Dark/quiet	=	Usually	=	3
Too hard/too soft	=	Not Usually	=	3
Getting to sleep	=	Sometimes	=	2
Back to sleep	=	Usually	=	1
Up at same time	=	Usually	=	4
Up naturally	=	Usually	=	3
Still tired	=	Not Usually	=	3
Sleep you need	=	Usually	=	4
		Total	=	36
Total ÷ 12	=	Sleep Score	=	3.00
		Grade	=	A

RELAXATION

Table 6.6

Question	Not Usually	Sometimes	Usually	Score
Do you have headaches?	3	2	1	_____
Do you easily get angry?	3	2	1	_____
Do you easily get anxious?	3	2	1	_____
Is it difficult for you to concentrate?	3	2	1	_____
Is it easy for you to laugh?	1	2	3	_____
Do coworkers think you are in a good mood?	1	2	3	_____
Do you feel energetic?	1	2	3	_____
Do you practice relaxation techniques or do *easy* aerobic exercises?	1	2	4	_____
			Total	_____
			Total ÷ 8	_____

Relaxation Score

In the Relaxation segment, round off to two decimal places.

Your Relaxation Score = _____

Table 6.7

Relaxation Grade	Range
A	2.89 – 3.13
B	2.39 – 2.88
C	1.64 – 2.38
D	1.14 – 1.63
F	1.00 – 1.13

Example:

Marlene

Headaches	=	Sometimes	=	2
Angry	=	Sometimes	=	2
Anxious	=	Sometimes	=	2
Hard to concentrate	=	Not Usually	=	3
Easy to laugh	=	Usually	=	3
Good mood	=	Usually	=	3
Energetic	=	Usually	=	3
Relaxation techniques	=	Not Usually	=	1
		Total	=	19
Total ÷ 8	=	Relaxation Score	=	2.38
		Grade	=	C

Dick

Headaches	=	Not Usually	=	3
Angry	=	Not Usually	=	3
Anxious	=	Not Usually	=	3
Hard to concentrate	=	Sometimes	=	2
Easy to laugh	=	Usually	=	3
Good mood	=	Usually	=	3

Energetic	=	Usually	=	3
Relaxation techniques	=	Sometimes	=	2
		Total	=	22
Total ÷ 8 =		Relaxation Score	=	2.75
		Grade	=	B

NUTRITION

There are people who feel that a complete dietary analysis is required to determine how diet affects you. While a complete professional analysis may be ideal, we have found that it is difficult to obtain an accurate analysis because of all the confounding factors such as agreement on composition of food, measurement of quantity of food, and ability to record food intake accurately and consistently. Therefore L.E.A.P. has questions of a more general nature that are designed to depict nutritional patterns and attitudes. We came to the conclusion that this overview is quite accurate in reflecting the role diet plays in your ability to convert energy.

Table 6.8

Question	Usually	Sometimes	Not Usually	Score
Do you eat fresh vegetables each day?	4	2	1	_____
Do you eat fresh fruit each day?	4	2	1	_____
Do you eat some legumes (beans, seeds, or sprouts) each day?	3	2	1	_____
Do you eat nutritious grains each day?	3	2	1	_____
If you are not allergic, do you consume some, but not too many, dairy products each day? If allergic, do you get calcium from another source?	3	2	1	_____
Do you eat some meat, but not too much, or get protein from another source, each day?	3	2	1	_____
Do you try to buy organic/chemical-free food?	3	2	1	_____
Are labels important in selecting what you eat?	3	2	1	_____
Do you try to buy mostly fresh foods as opposed to processed?	3	2	1	_____
In preparing foods, do you try to maintain nutritional value and minimize detrimental ingredients?	3	2	1	_____
Do you try to minimize fast food?	3	2	1	_____
Do you try to minimize junk food?	3	2	1	_____
Do you try minimize caffeine-based drinks?	3	2	1	
Are you a moderate or nondrinker?	Yes = 3	1	- 2	_____
Are you a nonsmoker?	Yes = 3	0	- 3	_____
			Total	_____
			Total ÷ 15	_____

Nutrition Score

In the Nutrition segment, round off to two decimal places.
Your Nutrition Score = _____

Table 6.9

Nutrition Grade	Range
A	2.81 – 3.13
B	2.21 – 2.80
C	1.28 – 2.20
D	0.74 – 1.27
F	0.53 – 0.73

Example:

Marlene

Vegetables	=	Sometimes	=	2
Fruits	=	Usually	=	4
Legumes	=	Sometimes	=	2
Grains	=	Usually	=	3
Dairy	=	Sometimes	=	2
Meats	=	Sometimes	=	2
Organic	=	Sometimes	=	2
Labels impt	=	Usually	=	3
Fresh	=	Usually	=	3
Prepare well	=	Sometimes	=	2
Minimize fast food	=	Usually	=	3
Minimize junk food	=	Usually	=	3
Minimize caffeine	=	Not Usually	=	1
Moderate alcohol	=	Yes	=	3
Nonsmoker	=	Yes	=	3
		Total	=	38
Total ÷ 15	=	Nutrition Score	=	2.53
		Grade	=	B

Dick

Vegetables	=	Usually	=	4
Fruits	=	Usually	=	4
Legumes	=	Usually	=	3
Grains	=	Usually	=	3
Dairy	=	Usually	=	3
Meats	=	Sometimes	=	2
Organic	=	Usually	=	3
Labels impt	=	Usually	=	3
Fresh	=	Usually	=	3
Prepare well	=	Sometimes	=	2
Minimize fast food	=	Usually	=	3
Minimize junk food	=	Sometimes	=	2
Minimize caffeine	=	Usually	=	3
Moderate alcohol	=	Yes	=	3
Nonsmoker	=	Yes	=	3
		Total	=	44
Total ÷ 15	=	Nutrition Score	=	2.93
		Grade	=	A

CURRENT PHYSICAL ACTIVITY

Your current physical activity plays a significant role in determining how well you convert energy. Choose the activity category that most accurately describes your current status. At this point genetics will play a role in your score because not all of us can be world-class athletes. Then estimate the average number of days per week you are currently active and the average minutes per day that you are active on the days you are active. Finally, try your best to select a level that represents the average intensity you feel when you are active. No one can do workouts that average above 85% VO2Max. You may be able to do steady state workouts day after day that are about 85% VO2Max. If you want help determining intensity level, go to Chapter 3 or Appendix C, How to Estimate Your Intensity. There, in addition to numbers that represent the intensity of the challenge, you will be given word clues to the difficulty of breathing and talking at various intensities.

Remember that activities that don't fit the classical idea of exercise can contribute to converting energy. So if you garden, walk on your job, or do housework or manual labor, these activities count.

Table 6.10

Value	Category	Days/Week	Minutes/Day	Intensity (%VO2Max)	Value
6	National/World-Class Competitor	7	> 90	85 Strong+	6
5.5	College Competitor	6	75-90	80	5.5
5	Adult Competitor	5	60-75	75 Strong	5
4.5	Active Adult	4	50-60	70	4.5
4	HS Competitor	3	40-50	65 Somewhat Strong	4
3.5	Age Group Competitor	2	30-40	60	3.5
3	Somewhat Active Young Adult	1	20-30	55 Moderate	3
2.5	Somewhat Active Student	Seasonal + Sporadic	15–20	50	2.5
2	Somewhat Active Adult	Better Than Sporadic	10-15	45 Easy	2
1.5	In Rehab	Sporadic	1-10	40 Very Easy	1.5
1	Inactive	Inactive	0	Nothing At All	1
	Category Score	Day/Week Score	Minute Score	Intensity Score	
	___	___	___	___	

Total Score ___
Total Score ÷ 4 ___

Current Physical Activity

You have 4 items to score in this table. Choose your answer for each item then record the value that goes with your selection. See the examples if you need help.

In the Current Physical Activity segment, round off to two decimal places.

Your Current Physical Activity Score = ___

Table 6.11

Activity Grade*	Range
A	5.51 – 6.00
B	4.26 – 5.50
C	2.51 – 4.25
D	1.26 – 2.50
F	1.00 – 1.25

*A grade of A is usually consistent with high-level endurance athletes

Example:

Marlene

Category	=	Active Adult	=	4.5
Days/Week	=	5	=	5.0
Minutes/Day	=	75–90	=	5.5
Intensity (%VO2Max)	=	50	=	2.5
		Total	=	17.5
		Total ÷ 4	=	4.38
		Grade	=	B

Dick

Category	=	Active Adult	=	4.5
Days/Week	=	5	=	5.0
Minutes/Day	=	50–60	=	4.5
Intensity (%VO2Max)	=	75	=	5.0
		Total	=	19
		Total ÷ 4	=	4.75
		Grade	=	B

ENERGY CONVERSION NUMBER

Now L.E.A.P. can begin to work its very precise magic. By turning all of these factors into an Energy Conversion Number, you are in a position to isolate and apply your own unique VO2Max to a customized program for yourself. Enter each score in the Table 6.12, and add them together to get your Energy Conversion Number. The Energy Conversion Number is a numerical representation of your ability to convert energy. Don't worry about how it compares to other people; this is a realistic estimate of where you are now. Nor should you worry about where you are now but focus just like with the grades, on another realistic fact—you can improve!

Table 6.12

Segment	Score
Age Score	_____
Pregnancy Score (if applicable)	_____
Fat-Free Weight Score	_____
Sleep Score	_____
Relaxation Score	_____
Nutrition Score	_____
Current Physical Activity Score	_____
Total	_____

Energy Conversion Number

Your Energy Conversion Number = _____

Example:

Marlene

Age Score	=	2
Pregnancy Score	=	0
Fat-Free Weight Score	=	4
Sleep Score	=	2.33
Relaxation Score	=	2.38
Nutrition Score	=	2.53
Current Physical Activity Score	=	4.38
Energy Conversion Number	=	17.62

Dick

Age Score	=	2
Pregnancy Score	=	0
Fat-Free Weight Score	=	4
Sleep Score	=	3
Relaxation Score	=	2.75
Nutrition Score	=	2.93
Physical Activity Score	=	4.75
Energy Conversion Number	=	19.43

No matter what your Energy Conversion Number is now, remember that it represents a point on a constantly changing health continuum. It won't change rapidly, but it will never be at the same point, even 24 hours from now. It simply shows your position on the health continuum at this particular time in your life. Look at it as a snapshot of where you stand today. It is indicative of how much energy you are able to safely convert by being physically active.

The score should provide hope and incentive to improve if you got a low score. It should make you feel good about yourself and determined to stay where you are if you got a high score. If you got a mid-range it means that you can improve your score by paying just a little more attention to the factors that contribute to your Energy Conversion Number.

What else does your Energy Conversion Number mean? First, it provides a basis for starting or continuing a physical activity program at the level that is exactly right for you. Second, it gives you a very good idea of how you would score on common fitness tests. Your overall fitness should be able to be described in the same terms as your ability to convert energy. If you have a high energy conversion grade, you are very likely to have a high grade in a most useful and important fitness test, VO2Max.

VO2MAX

VO2Max is an indication of your maximum ability to remove oxygen from the air, transfer it to the blood, deliver it to the cells, and use it for energy conversion. Since most of the energy converted in your cells is derived from the combination of oxygen with the end product of carbohydrate, fat, and protein fuels, the ability to use oxygen is crucial to the cells that make up your body. Other things being equal, the more oxygen you can use, the better your health.

In the next table you will be able to find the VO2Max that is closest to your actual energy conversion ability. This table is large, but it's simple to use. All you have to do is find your Energy Conversion Number, and that will tell you your VO2Max. You will use your VO2Max to find out exactly how much physical activity is right for you.

Find the Energy Conversion Number that is closest to yours. In the column to the right of that number is your VO2Max.

Table 6.15

Conversion Number	VO2Max	Conversion Number	VO2Max	Conversion Number	VO2Max
23.51	72	18.92	49	9.30	26
23.39	71	18.59	48	8.97	25
23.28	70	18.26	47	8.64	24
23.16	69	17.93	46	8.31	23
23.05	68	17.46	45	7.98	22
22.93	67	17.00	44	7.66	21
22.82	66	16.53	43	7.33	20
22.70	65	16.06	42	7.00	19
22.58	64	15.60	41	6.67	18
22.47	63	15.13	40	6.34	17
22.35	62	14.66	39	6.02	16
22.24	61	14.19	38	5.69	15
22.12	60	13.73	37	5.36	14
22.01	59	13.26	36		
21.89	58	12.80	35		
21.56	57	12.33	34		
21.23	56	11.87	33		
20.90	55	11.40	32		
20.57	54	10.94	31		
20.24	53	10.61	30		
19.91	52	10.28	29		
19.58	51	9.95	28		
19.25	50	9.62	27		

Energy Conversion Number and VO2Max

Your VO2Max = _____ ml/kg/min

Example:

Marlene

Energy Conversion Numbers   =   17.62

VO2Max   =   45 ml/kg/min

Dick

Energy Conversion Numbers   =   19.43

VO2Max   =   50 ml/kg/min

Remember, the units for VO2Max are milliliters per kilograms of body weight per minute. In other words, VO2Max measures the maximum milliliters of oxygen you can use in a minute for every kilogram you weigh.

I put the amount of oxygen used in terms of soft drink cans per minute because I have found that people can see this in their minds. You can find the total number of soft drink cans of oxygen you can use per minute by using the formula below:

Soft Drink Cans of Oxygen/Min = VO2Max (ml/kg/min) x 1 Can/350 ml x Weight (lb)/2.2 lb/kg

     = .0013 x Your VO2Max x Your Weight

     = .0013 x _____ x _____ = _____ Cans /Min

Example:

Marlene

Cans/Min.   =   .0013 x 45 x 143   =   8.4 cans/min

Dick

Cans/Min.   =   .0013 x 50 x 194   =   12.6 cans/min

The amount of oxygen I can use is higher than Marlene's primarily because I am heavier. Corrected for weight, I only use 8% more oxygen per minute. But that 8% difference does mean I convert oxygen somewhat more efficiently, and it would make a difference in performance. If we were to both run a mile, I would probably beat her by 25 seconds.

If I wanted to improve my VO_{2Max} from 50 to 51, I could raise my Energy Conversion Number from 19.43 to 19.58. Increasing physical activity is not the only way I could do this. If I were to be a little more careful about junk food, keep the bedroom quieter, and practice a little more relaxation technique I could raise my Energy Conversion Number.

Increasing your ability to use oxygen will help you convert energy efficiently, and that means moving forward on the health continuum and increasing your performance.

You are now ready to use your VO_{2Max}, and let L.E.A.P. show you how. L.E.A.P. does it by answering a very practical question: "How much physical activity should I do my first week?"

CHAPTER 7

WEEK 1 OPTIMAL ENERGY CONVERSION POINTS

SUPPORT AND TIME

While support and time may not directly affect metabolic rate, they are nevertheless important. It turns out that support enhances a person's ability to participate in physical activity. The better the support, the more likely you are to convert energy through physical activity.

Time, a major excuse many people give for not being physically active, also plays a role. My friend Dan had a consistent L.E.A.P. Log in which he documented that week after week he met his optimal level of physical activity. Then his wife gave birth to two beautiful children within 2½ years. To say the least, this affected Dan's ability to be as physically active as he was. For a few years he is going to have to be satisfied with less physical activity, but with the L.E.A.P. program he will be able to keep physical activity in his life at a level he knows is producing healthy, if not optimal, benefits.

Table 7.1

Question	Usually	Sometimes	Not Usually	Score
Do you make physical activity as important as any other item on your calendar?	4	2	1	_____
Does your partner share or support your physical activity? (2 if not applicable)	4	2	1	_____
Do your family/friends share or support your physical activity?	3	2	1	_____
Does your employer support your physical activity? (2 if not applicable)	3	2	1	_____
Do you work 40 hours per week or less?	3	2	1	_____
Do you spend less than 4 hours a week on other obligations, such as school, church, clubs?	3	2	1	_____
If you live with children, does it help make you more physically active? (3 if not applicable)	3	2	1	_____
Do you watch less than 10 hours of TV/videos a week?	3	2	1	_____
			Total	_____
			Total ÷ 8	_____

Support/Time Score

Your Support/Time Score = ____

Table 7.2

Grade	Range
A	3.01 – 3.25
B	2.51 – 3.00
C	1.64 – 2.50
D	1.14 – 1.63
F	1.00 – 1.13

Example:

Marlene

Importance on calendar	=	Sometimes	=	2
Partner support	=	Usually	=	4
Family/friends support	=	Sometimes	=	2
Employer support	=	Not Usually	=	1
40-hour week	=	Not usually	=	1
Other obligations	=	Usually	=	3
Children	=	Not Applicable	=	3
10 hours TV	=	Sometimes	=	2
		Total	=	18
Support/Time Score		Total ÷ 8	=	2.25
		Grade	=	C

Dick

Importance on calendar	=	Usually	=	4
Partner support	=	Usually	=	4
Family/friends support	=	Usually	=	3
Employer support	=	Usually	=	3
40-hour week	=	Sometimes	=	2
Other obligations	=	Usually	=	3
Children	=	Not Applicable	=	3
10 hours TV	=	Not usually	=	1
		Total	=	23
Support/Time Score		Total ÷ 8	=	2.88
		Grade	=	B

DETERMINING YOUR WEEK 1
OPTIMAL ENERGY CONVERSION POINTS

As of now you have a very important number, your VO2Max, and you have a modifier of that number in the form of a Support/Time Score. It's now time to show you how to get your Week 1 Optimal Energy Conversion Points, which are the optimal number of points for you to earn during the first week of your program. I will refer to Energy Conversion Points as ECPs, pronounced as the letters *E-C-Ps*. Your Week 1 Optimal ECPs represent exactly the right place for you to start your L.E.A.P. program. The units for ECPs are points, but they also represent liters of oxygen consumed per week in physical activity. Your Week 1 Optimal ECPs are the number of liters of oxygen you are capable of consuming during physical activity in the first week on the L.E.A.P. program. ECPs can approximate calories if you multiply the ECPs by 4.85.

Week 1 Optimal ECPs, the goal for your first week on the L.E.A.P. program, allow you wide ranges of energy conversion for individual workouts but keep you within your weekly ability to convert energy.

L.E.A.P. arrives at this starting number by combining:

- A suggested frequency, duration, and intensity of your weekly physical activities
- Your Support/Time Score, modified by the perfect Support/Time Score
- The conversion of all metric units to English units
- A number representing your VO2Max called the VO2Max Coefficient
- Your weight

FREQUENCY, DURATION, INTENSITY

Frequency is easy to determine. It is how many times you are active in a week.

Duration is also easy to determine. It is how many minutes you are active whenever you do a physical activity.

Intensity, which is closely tied to VO2Max, can be more difficult to determine. Scientists spend time effort, and money doing experiments to determine what percentage of your VO2Max you are using or how many calories are converted during an activity. Is there a general way to determine intensity that is acceptable to both the lay public and the scientific community?

The answer is yes. Estimating intensity can be almost as easy as determining duration. We can do this because of Borg's work with rating of perceived exertion (RPE). RPE was discussed in Chapter 3, and a further discussion can be found in Appendix C.

By way of review, in the early 1960s Dr. Gunnar Borg began working to determine if people could accurately assess their intensity level because he realized that intensity measurements were not available to the public. He had measured people on scientific equipment, but he wondered if they could accurately estimate the intensity at which they worked. By measuring their intensity (%VO2Max) and at the same time asking them to select numbers and phrases that described that intensity, he established that most people could make an accurate estimate of how hard they were working.

He developed scales that tied numbers and words to intensity levels. These scales are used worldwide in clinics and in research. The RPE scale used and modified by L.E.A.P. was developed by Dr. Borg and his associate Dr. Bruce Noble and is a 10-point scale. For clarity, I have substituted synonyms for some of the words. I have also found that the use of additional word descriptions makes it easier for different people to relate to the scales. For example, some people are more in tune with their breathing, others with their ability to talk during physical activity.

From Chapter 3 you may recall that there is an Intensity Coefficient (I$_{coef}$) that is associated with each estimate of perceived effort. In determining your Week 1 Optimal ECPs, L.E.A.P. combines the appropriate Intensity Coefficient with a frequency and duration goal that is consistent with the activity category you selected in your autobiography.

The next several paragraphs may seem mundane, but I want you to understand how L.E.A.P. generates numbers that are valuable to you. So either bear with them or skip them, but know they are there because I don't want to hide processes from you.

Based upon what I have formally learned on my way to a Ph.D. and upon what I have observed in 35 years of helping people perform or make activity a part of their lives, I have combined some of the variables that determine Week 1 Optimal ECPs into another number, the Week 1 Coefficient. By doing this I have made it much easier for you to calculate your starting points. Several factors contribute to the Week 1 Coefficient. One, as you know, is a number associated with your activity category and represents the frequency, duration, and intensity per week that are reasonable for you to aspire to.

I multiply frequency times duration times intensity and modify that by dividing three more numbers that I call unit conversion numbers into the product. One number converts milliliters to liters. A second converts pounds to kilograms. The third modifies your Support/Time Score, converting it to a fraction of the the maximum Support/Time Score possible.

All of this sounds complex, but it will give you a single number, the Week 1 Coefficient(W1$_{coef}$), which:

1. Means you don't have to do a lot of math when you determine your Week 1 Optimal ECPs
2. Will give you a number that represents liters of oxygen to be consumed per week in physical activity.

Table 7.3 shows the results of the math and the coefficient you will use for your Week 1 Optimal ECPs. Appendix O shows an example of the steps I took to get the final coefficient.

Find the Activity Category you selected in your autobiograpy. In the column to its right is the Week 1 Coefficient (W1Coef) you will use.

Table 6.3

Activity Category	Week 1 Coefficient
National/WC Competitor	.141
College Competitor	.116
Adult Competitor	.082
HS Competitor	.057
Active Adult	.047
Age group Competitor	.032
Somewhat Active Young Adult	.023
Somewhat Active Student	.019
Somewhat Active Adult	.017
In Rehabilitation	.009
Inactive	.004

Week 1 Coefficent

Your Week 1 Coefficient = _____

Example:

Marlene

Activity Category = Active Adult

W1Coef = .047

Dick

Activity Category = Active Adult

W1Coef = .047

VO$_2$MAX COEFFICIENT

A number representing your VO$_2$Max will also be used to determine your Week 1 Optimal ECPs. This number has also been modified from your VO$_2$Max to account for the exponential character of energy conversion as VO$_2$Max and %VO$_2$Max change.

Find your VO$_2$Max in Table 7.4. In the column to its right is your VO$_2$Max Coefficient.

Table 7.4

VO_2Max	$VO_2Max<$ Coef	VO_2Max	VO_2Max Coef	VO_2Max	VO_2Max Coef
72	42.86	52	26.51	32	12.94
71	41.99	51	25.76	31	12.35
70	41.12	50	25.01	30	11.76
69	40.25	49	24.28	29	11.19
68	39.39	48	23.55	28	10.62
67	38.54	47	22.83	27	10.07
66	37.69	46	22.12	26	9.52
65	36.85	45	21.41	25	8.99
64	36.02	44	20.71	24	8.46
63	35.19	43	20.02	23	7.94
62	34.37	42	19.33	22	7.44
61	33.55	41	18.66	21	6.95
60	32.74	40	17.99	20	6.46
59	31.94	39	17.33	19	5.99
58	31.15	38	16.68	18	5.53
57	30.36	37	16.03	17	5.08
56	29.57	36	15.40	16	4.65
55	28.80	35	14.77	15	4.23
54	28.03	34	14.15	14	3.82
53	27.26	33	13.54		

VO_2Max Coefficent

Your VO_2Max Coefficient = _____

Example:

Marlene

VO_2Max = 45

VO_2Max Coef = 21.41

Dick

VO_2Max = 50

VO_2Max Coef = 25.01

With your W1Coef and VO_2MaxCoef it is easy to get your Week 1 Optimal ECPs. You don't have to worry about terms. All you have to do is multiply four numbers together:

Week 1 Optimal ECPs = W1Coef x VO_2MaxCoef x Support/Time Score x Weight

Example:

Marlene

W1Coef = .047

VO_2MaxCoef = 21.41

Support/Time Score = 2.25

Weight = 143

Now to get her Week 1 Optimal ECPs, all Marlene has to do is multiply those four numbers:

Week 1 Optimal ECPs = .047 x 21.41 x 2.25 x 143 = 324

During the first week Marlene is on the L.E.A.P. program, her optimal goal is to earn 324 ECPs by consuming 324 liters of oxygen in physical activities.

Dick

Week 1 Optimal ECPs = .047 x 25.01 x 2.88 x 194 = 657

YOUR WEEK 1 OPTIMAL ECPS CONVERSION POINTS

Now you can determine the place to start that is exactly right for you. Very few other people will have your exact Week 1 Optimal ECPs, and if they do, they will have arrived at them through totally different numbers. These Week 1 Optimal ECPs belong to you.

Step 1.

Your Week 1 Coef = _____
Your Vo2MaxCoef = _____
Your Support/Time Score = _____
Your Weight = _____

Step 2. *Multiply those four values.*
Step 3. *Your Week 1 Optimal ECPs* = _____ *ECPs or Liters O2/wk*

L.E.A.P. uses points and liters interchangeably. They both end up meaning the same thing. They represent how much energy you can convert through physical activity each week.

If you want to find out how many soft drink cans of oxygen your ECPs represent, divide by 0.35.

Example:

Marlene
Soft Drink Cans of O2/Wk   =   324 L/.35 L per can = 926

Dick
Soft Drink Cans of O2/Wk   =   657 L/.35 L per Can = 1877

You now have your Week 1 Optimal ECPs. This is an important number. It's your optimal energy conversion number for week 1. You can now use that number to develop a plan.

CHAPTER 8

LEVELS AND ZONES

*L*et's take a closer look at the Week 1 Optimal ECPs and use them to develop a plan. The number you have now represents the optimal amount of oxygen you should consume in physical activity for the first week. To put it another way, it is the amount of energy you should convert by physical activity to challenge your body enough to optimally improve but not so much that you enter Selye's exhaustion stage.

How do you meet this goal? You get credit for all physical activities you do. What I will do now is show you how to figure ECPs for each physical activity you do. To do this, you simply need to be able to multiply three numbers: your VO2MaxWeight Coefficient, duration, and intensity.

To get your VO2MaxWeight Coefficient you multiply the VO2MaxCoef from the last chapter by your weight and divide by 1936.

VO2MaxWgtCoef = VO2MaxCoef x Weight ÷ 1936

Now determine your VO2MaxWgtCoef.

Your VO2MaxCoef = _____
Your Weight = _____
Your VO2MaxWgtCoef · = _____ x _____ ÷1936 =

_____

Example:

Marlene

VO2MaxCoef   =   21.41

Weight   =   143

VO2MaxWgtCoef   =   21.41 x 143 ÷ 1936 = 1.58

Dick

VO2MaxCoef   =   25.01

Weight   =   194

VO2MaxWgtCoef   =   25.01 x 194 ÷ 1936 = 2.51

If your VO2Max or weight change, you can get a new VO2MaxWgtCoef. Using the VO2MaxWgtCoef saves you time when you determine your ECPs.

The number 1936 is used to convert milliliters to liters and pounds to kilograms. Normally the number would be 2200 because there are 1000 ml in a liter and 2.2 pounds in a kilogram. I have used regression equations to modify this to 1936 to account for the exponential effect of VO2Max, intensity, duration, and other individual factors.

Now you are ready to figure out how many ECPs you earn from a single bout of physical activity. You already have your VO2MaxWgtCoef.

Duration is how long you were active.

Intensity is how hard your activity was. You determine your intensity by using the Modified Borg-Noble Intensity Scale, which is shown in Table 8.1.

Table 8.1

RPE	Challenge was	Breathing was	Talking was	%VO2Max	ICoef
1.0	Very Easy	Normal	Normal	35	0.08
1.5				40	0.16
2.0	Easy	Normal	Normal	45	0.26
2.5				50	0.37
3.0	Moderate	Comfortable	Easy	55	0.51
3.5				60	0.66
4.0	Somewhat Strong	Noticeable	Somewhat Difficult	65	0.82
4.5				70	1.00
5.0	Strong	Deep, but Steady	Difficult	75	1.20
5.5				80	1.40
6.0	Between Strong & Very Strong	Deep & Somewhat Rapid	Between Difficult & Very Difficult	85	1.62
6.5				87.5	1.86
7.0	Very Strong	Deep & Rapid	Very Difficult	90	2.10
7.5				92.5	2.36
8.0	Very, Very Strong	Very Deep & Very Rapid	Extremely Difficult	95	2.63
8.5				96.1	2.91
9.0				97.5	3.21
9.5				98.8	3.51
10	Maximum Effort	Breathlessness	Impossible	100	3.83

Modified Borg-Noble Intensity Scale

Here's a Marlene example. I'm going to put it in bold print this time because it is the process you will do every time you are physically active.

Example:

Let's say Marlene walked for 30 minutes at an intensity that was between easy and moderate (her breathing was normal to comfortable, and talking was normal to easy). This level of exertion correlates to an RPE of 2.5 and an intensity of 50% VO2Max on the Modified Borg-Noble Intensity Scale. The Intensity Coefficient (ICoef) is 0.37.

$$\text{Marlene}$$
$$\text{VO2MaxWgtCoef} = 1.58$$
$$\text{Duration} = 30 \text{ minutes}$$
$$\text{ICoef} = .37$$
$$\text{ECPs} = (1.58 \times 30 \times .37) = 18$$

Since Marlene's Week 1 Optimal ECPs are 324, she has accomplished 6% of her goal and has 306 ECPs remaining for the week.

$$\text{Dick}$$
For the same duration and intensity Dick earns 28 ECPs.
$$2.51 \times 30 \times .37 = \quad 28$$

Now, figure out your ECPs if you were active for 30 minutes at 50% VO2Max.

Your VO2MaxWgtCoef = _____
Duration = 30 minutes
ICoef = .37
ECPs = _____

Figuring out your ECPs each time you are active is very easy. Just multiply your VO2MaxWgtCoef x Duration x ICoef.

Now multiply the ECPs number you just got by 7.

ECPs x 7 = _____

Example:

Marlene

ECPs = 18

18 x 7 = 126

Dick

ECPs = 28

28 x 7 = 196

When Marlene earns 126 ECPs and Dick earns 196 ECPs in a week, they reach their Disease Risk Reduction Level. What you just figured out was your Disease Risk Reduction Level. When you earn this many ECPs in a week, your physical activity is reducing your risk of degenerative diseases. If your Week 1 Optimal ECPs are not that high now, do not try to reach this level. In the next chapter L.E.A.P. will show you how to build up to that level slowly.

The disease risk reduction level is one of the levels of success L.E.A.P. has built into your program.

LEVELS

At this point you know what your optimal goal is for the first week, your Week 1 Optimal ECPs. You also know how to compute your ECPs for each physical activity. Now I can tell you about the safe minimum level, the risk reduction level, the body change level, the VO2Max change level, the optimal level, and the overtraining level.

With the exception of the last two levels, the American Medical Association, the American College of Sports Medicine, and the Office of the Surgeon General have all recently published physical activity guidelines and benefits that accrue by reaching various levels of physical activity. L.E.A.P. has translated those guidelines and levels to ECPs that relate to you as an individual. The levels and their benefits are shown below:

Level	Benefit
Safe Minimum	This is a safe minimum starting level for someone who is inactive and has a low VO2Max.
Risk Reduction	Chronic degenerative disease risk is reduced.
Body Change	Fat weight decreases and fat-free weight increases.
VO2Max Change	VO2Max improves.
Optimal	Your energy conversion is just right for you. You are getting maximum benefits from physical activity.
Overtraining	You are doing too much. This will result in an increased risk of illness, injury, or burnout.

Each level is associated with a frequency, duration, and intensity, and ECPs can be related to each level. Find your levels by multiplying your VO2MaxWgtCoef, by the appropriate guidelines, as follows:

$Level = VO_{2MaxWgtCoef} \times Frequency^* \times Duration \times I_{Coef}$

$Safe\ Minimum\ =\ \underline{\hspace{1.5cm}} \times 7 \times 10 \times .26\ =\ \underline{\hspace{1.5cm}}$

$Risk\ Reduction\ =\ \underline{\hspace{1.5cm}} \times 7 \times 30 \times .37\ =\ \underline{\hspace{1.5cm}}$

$Body\ Change\ =\ \underline{\hspace{1.5cm}} \times 4 \times 30 \times .82\ =\ \underline{\hspace{1.5cm}}$

$VO_{2Max}\ Change\ =\ \underline{\hspace{1.5cm}} \times 4 \times 40 \times .82\ =\ \underline{\hspace{1.5cm}}$

$Optimal\ =\ Week\ 1\ Optimal\ ECPs\ =\ \underline{\hspace{1.5cm}}$

$Overtraining\ =\ Optimal \times 1.075\ =\ \underline{\hspace{1.5cm}}$

* Frequency is how many times per week you do this.

Example:

	Marlene	
Safe Minimum =	1.58 x 7 x 10 x .26 =	29
Risk Reduction =	1.58 x 7 x 30 x .37 =	123[1]
Body Change =	1.58 x 4 x 30 x .82 =	156
VO2Max Change =	1.58 x 4 x 40 x .82 =	207
Optimal =	324	
Overtraining =	Optimal x 1.075 =	348

If Marlene were inactive, with all other characteristics the same, she could start a physical activity program at a safe level of 29 ECPs. That's 10 minutes a day at about 45% VO2Max. She will reduce her risk of degenerative diseases if she attains 123 ECPs, will improve her muscle-to-fat ratio if she attains 156 ECPs, and will begin to improve her VO2Max when she gets to 207. If she reaches 324 she is doing the best she can for her body at the present time. If she goes over 348 she will enter the early stages of Selye's exhaustion stage and will run a greater risk of illness, injury, or burnout. Being at her overtraining level is not good and will lead to a pattern of inconsistent activiy.

---

[1] The 123 instead of 126 is due to rounding off of 17.538 to 18 in previous example.

Example:

Dick

Safe Minimum	=	2.51 x 7 x 10 x .26	= 46
Risk Reduction	=	2.51 x 7 x 30 x .37	= 196
Body Change	=	2.51 x 4 x 30 x .82	= 247
VO2Max Change	=	2.51 x 4 x 40 x .82	= 329
Optimal	=	657	
Overtraining	=	Optimal x 1.075	= 706

Levels are another way L.E.A.P. helps guide you toward making physical activity a consistent, successful factor in your life.

ZONES

L.E.A.P. has also established three zones in which you can reside with respect to physical activity: the success zone, the optimal zone, and the overtraining zone.

The *success zone* begins when you exceed your risk reduction level and continues up to 92.5% of your optimal level. In this zone you are doing enough physical activity to make it beneficial and are probably doing more than what 80% of the rest of America is doing.

You get into the *optimal zone* when you attain more than 92.5% but less than 107.5% of your optimal level. In this zone you are doing exactly what is right for you. Your optimal level, which represents energy conversion at a level that is best for your body right now, is at the center of the optimal zone. As you get near the optimal level you can play "What if?" to get as close as possible to that number. You don't have to hit the number exactly, so don't get picky about it.

If you go over 107.5% of your optimal level, you are in the *overtraining zone*. Your body will say "Ouch!" You may be able to get away with doing this for a few weeks, but very soon you will enter Selye's exhaustion stage and no longer be able to be physically active because of illness, injury, or burnout.

You should find out what your zones are.

You already figured out the low end of your success zone, which is your risk reduction level.

Your risk reduction level = _____ECPs.

Example:

Marlene

Risk Reduction = 123 ECPs

Dick

Risk Reduction = 196 ECPs

High End of Your Success Zone = .925 x Week 1 Optimal ECPs = _____ECPs

Your Overtraining Zone = 1.075 x Week 1 Optimal ECPs = _____ECPs

Example:

Marlene

High End Success Zone = 324 x .925   = 300 ECPs
Overtraining Zone = 324 x 1.075 = 348 ECPs

Dick

High End Success Zone = 657 x .925   = 608ECPs
Overtraining Zone = 657 x 1.075 = 706 ECPs

Now you know some levels and zones that can help you with your physical activity program. You know that even if you don't reach your optimal goal, physical activity can still make a beneficial difference. We expect everybody, even those of us who wrote this program, to exercise in the success zone from time to time because everyone has a grandma who visits them once in a while.

Now let's take a look at a table of the zones to see how they all fit together. If your optimal level is below the risk reduction level, you should not concern yourself with zones. Instead just focus on reaching your optimal level and progressing slowly to a point in your program where your optimal level is higher than your risk reduction level. In the next chapter, L.E.A.P. will show you how to make progress, and in a moment you'll see what your zone table looks like.

Example:

Marlene

Table 8.2

	≥ 123	≥ 300	> 348
	Success Zone	**Optimal Zone**	**Overtraining Zone**
Safe Minimum = 29	Body Change = 156	Optimal = 324	
Risk Reduction = 123	VO2Max Change = 207		

Dick

Table 8.3

	≥ 196	≥ 608	> 706
	Success Zone	**Optimal Zone**	**Overtraining Zone**
Safe Minimum = 46	Body Change = 247	Optimal = 657	
Risk Reduction = 196	VO2Max Change = 329		

In these examples the optimal level was higher than any other level. In other cases the optimal level could be lower than risk reduction, body change, or VO2Max change. If this happens with you, all levels that are higher than the optimal level should be placed in the appropriate zone, as shown in the example below.

Table 8.4

	≥ 123	≥ 194	> 226
	Success Zone	**Optimal Zone**	**Overtraining Zone**
Safe Minimum = 29	Body Change = 156	Optimal = 210	
Risk Reduction = 123		VO2Max Change = 218	

In the next example the optimal level is lower than the risk reduction level. This person is starting at the safe minimum—10 minutes a day at an intensity of 45% VO2Max.

Table 8.5

		≥ 27	> 31
	Success Zone	**Optimal Zone**	**Overtraining Zone**
Safe Minimum = 29		Optimal = 29	Risk Reduction = 123
			Body Change = 137
			VO2Max Change = 151

In this example there is no success zone until reaching the optimal zone. In addition to proceeding as suggested in the next chapter, a person in this situation should redo the autobiography every two or three weeks because by virtue of changing from an inactive person to a somewhat active or active person, the Energy Conversion Number will increase dramatically, allowing for more rapid progress. Just starting with a 10-minute L.E.A.P. will get you to a higher level sooner than you think.

Now using your levels and zones fill out Table 8.6.

Table 8.6

	Success Zone	Optimal Zone	Overtraining Zone
Safe Minimum = _____			

First fill in the beginning of your success zone, then the beginning of the optimal zone, and then the beginning of the overtraining zone.

Second, fill in the levels (risk reduction, body change, VO2Max change, and optimal) in the zone in which they fit as shown in the earlier examples.

Here are a few more general concepts that you should remember about L.E.A.P. and ECPs.

ECPs don't need to be accomplished by doing physical activity a specified number of days every week. Some weeks you can do fewer days, others more. You can choose the days.

ECPs don't have to be accomplished by doing physical activity a specified number of minutes. Some days you may want to do fewer minutes, some days more. You can choose the duration.

ECPs don't have to be accomplished by always working at the same level of intensity. Some efforts can be easier, some harder. You can choose the intensity.

ECPs don't have to be accomplished by doing the same activity day after day unless you really enjoy that activity. You can choose the activities.

It's very beneficial to have variety in frequency, duration, intensity, and type of activity. With ECPs you can have variety in all of those areas.

All you need to do with ECPs is try to attain your goal. At the end of the week, the ECPs should come close to your optimal goal for the week. Here is another example from Marlene and myself.

Example:

Marlene

Optimal Goal = 324 ECPs

	Duration (min)	I_{Coef}	ECPs
Sunday*	60	.51	= 48
Monday	90	.26	= 37
Tuesday	80	.26	= 33
Wednesday	80	.26	= 33
Thursday	70	.37	= 41
Friday	55	.26	= 23
	30	.82	= 39
Saturday	50	.66	= 52
	Weekly Total		**= 306**
	Zone		= Optimal

*Marlene's job as an office nurse requires significant low-level physical activity. Marlene got her ECPs from the office work, walking, gardening, and housework.

Dick

Optimal Goal = 657 ECPs

	Duration (min)	I_{Coef}	ECPs
Sunday*	40	1.00	= 100
Monday	off		=
Tuesday	50	1.40	= 176
Wednesday	35	1.40	= 123

Thursday	50	1.00	=	126
Friday	off		=	
Saturday	30	1.86	=	140
	Weekly Total		**=**	**665**
	Zone		=	Optimal

*This was from the week of October 5, 1997. I got all my ECPs from the Concept II Rowing Machine.

One point that can be made from the two examples is that your physical activity can be very structured or very flexible. It's up to you, your schedule, and your interests.

You simply need to know your optimal level and try your best to earn that number of ECPs each week. If you fall short, you can still be in your success zone and benefit from reaching the risk reduction, body change, or VO2Max change level. L.E.A.P. makes it simple.

You could stop reading now and have a very good program concept. Reach you optimal level each week by multiplying three numbers together each time you are active:

VO2Max Wgtgcoef x duration x Icoef.

However, L.E.A.P. can make your program even better.

CHAPTER 9

THE SCHEDULES

Now that you know how many ECPs you can be earning on a weekly basis, how do you go about setting up a schedule for the week?

Remember, you have a lot of flexibility in how you can earn your ECPs each week. But some ways are better than others. For instance, you don't ever want to earn all your points on one day. You have determined how much energy you can convert in a week. If it is all spent in one day, it will overwhelm your resources. You may be able to do that one or two times, but you will soon find that you can't continue in this manner. You will stop being physically active. In fact, it is wise not to earn more than 40% of your weekly ECPs in one day.

What are some concepts that will help you develop a weekly plan? Several ideas have merit and have been used successfully for years in track. One of these, called "hard day–easy day," was developed by Bill Bowerman of the University of Oregon. He coached thirty-two Olympians and was one of the leaders of the worldwide jogging movement of the late '60s and early '70s. He felt that any hard day should be followed by an easy day. Easy days for some people can mean doing nothing and for others can mean a 6-mile run. Again, it depends upon your ability to convert energy.

Another concept was developed by Arthur Lydiard. He felt you could work out every day if your intensity was no greater than about 85% VO2Max. Staying below this intensity level means that you can recover within 24 hours. If you go too far above 85% VO2Max or stay there too long, recovery will probably take 48 hours or more.

The Table 9.1 provides a third way for you to divide up your weekly ECPs. The daily percentages are suggestions based upon several factors, including the thoughts of Mr. Bowerman and Mr. Lydiard and my own experience. Doing these percentages enables you to come back for more— weekly, monthly, and yearly. But remember not to get too concerned about hitting exact percentages. You can use the table as a general guide when you plan your activity.

Table 9.1

Days/ Week Active	Day 1	Day 2	Day 3	Day 4	Day 5	Day 6	Day 7
3	33		33		33		
4	30		22		26		22
5	26	12	20		22		20
6	24	12	16		20	12	16
7	22	10	15	10	18	10	15

Daily Percentages of Weekly ECPs

You can see from the table that you should plan to be physically active at least 3 days each week. Less than that and it is difficult to imagine that physical activity is really a part of your life. The maximum you should ever do on any one day is 40% of your optimal ECPs level.

If you don't want to follow a weekly percentage schedule, remember the hard day-easy day principle: follow any hard day with an easy day. Or remember the steady state principle: keep the intensity below 85% VO2Max.

It is my suggestion to make Sunday the first day of every workout week. This is to mentally separate the weekend. If you look at Monday as the first day of the workout week, there is a tendency to think that if you don't get your physical activity in during the week you can always pick it up on the weekend. This often results in 2 hard days back to back, which increases the risk of illness and injury. Also, if you need to do something else on the weekend, you have created a consistency problem. To make activity a part of your life, you must make it a part of your weekdays too. So develop that habit right from the start.

One of the useful things about ECPs and goals is that by Saturday you know exactly where you stand and can plan your workout so you get that number of points. Too often people figure they have more time on the weekends so they just do a lot and then wonder why they are more tired or not interested in physical activity during the week. ECPs give you the opportunity to fine-tune the physical activity that is right for you on the last workout day of the week.

For example, say that it's Saturday and your optimal level for the week is 500 ECPs. You planned to work out on Saturday but see that you have already earned 460 ECPs. You need only 40 more points to reach your level of 500. Instead of working out really hard and overshooting your goal, you know exactly what you need and can structure the workout accordingly. You can give yourself permission to work out at an easier pace than you may have thought. Your thinking should be, "If I am physically active for 10 minutes at 65% VO2Max I will get 40 ECPs and hit exactly 500 ECPs for the week."

On the other hand, if you need a lot of ECPs, you can work out with the knowledge that as long as you don't go over 40% of the weekly total, it's OK. Let's say your ECPs goal is 500 and you have accumulated only 200 ECPs through Friday night. You still need 300 more ECPs to reach your level. But 300 ECPs is more than 40% of 500; 40% of 500 is 200 ECPs. What should you do? You should earn 200 ECPs and be satisfied that you reached 400 for the week. If you go ahead and do 300, you will have reached the weekly goal at the risk of decreasing your chances of making physical activity a part of your life. Sometime during the next 2 weeks you would probably have to stop or feel you didn't want to continue. You would not know where the feeling came from. It would have come from overworking on the day you got 300 ECPs, or 60% of your weekly goal, in one day.

SETTING UP A 13-WEEK SCHEDULE

Obviously you don't want to stop physical activity after one week, so the next step is to set up a program that allows you to maintain or improve your level of energy conversion. L.E.A.P. gives you two options. The choice is up to you. If you are satisfied with your current level of physical activity and it results in ECPs equal to or greater than the risk reduction level, you can choose L.E.A.P.'s Maintenance Program. If you want to further improve your health, enjoy more physical activity, or perform better, L.E.A.P. suggests a Progression Program that daily, weekly, quarterly, and yearly balances challenge and recovery, enabling you to adapt to ever-increasing levels of physical activity. Both programs are based on 13-week cycles.

A 13-week cycle is a good choice for several reasons. First, chronologically it fits into the year nicely: 13 x 4 = 52. Second, and more important, abundant research has shown that physiologically measurable results occur in 10 to 12 weeks. Third, 13 weeks allow for additional recovery near the end of the 13-week period, solidifying adaptation.

MAINTENANCE PROGRAM

If you choose to maintain your current ECP level, you will maintain that level for 10 weeks.

In Week 11 you will reduce your ECPs to 75% of the

starting level. In Week 12 you will reduce your ECPs to 50% of the starting level. After Week 12 you take a week off, doing nothing or "active rest" at the most. The athletes I coach always ask me to define *active rest*. It's very simple. If during the time off period you feel you want to do something physical, ask yourself the question "Do I want to do this because it will be fun or because I feel I'm getting out of shape?" If the answer is "It will be fun," do it, do it at low intensity, and don't record it. Have fun! If the answer is "I'm getting out of shape," don't do the activity. Give your body, especially your endocrine system, a break. Taking the week off insures the balancing of long-term challenge and recovery so that adaptation is produced. The 13th week solidifies recovery and keeps you fresh.

If you chose the 13-week Maintenance Program, a graph of your weekly goals would look like this:

Figure 9.1

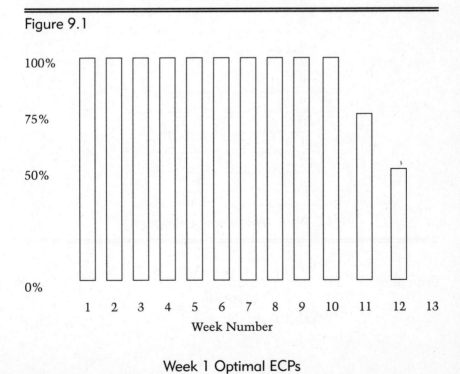

Week 1 Optimal ECPs

13-WEEK MAINTENANCE GRAPH

The Table 9.2 allows you to fill in ECPs for each of the 13 weeks in a Maintenance Program. Just put your Week 1 Optimal ECPs in the first 10 weeks. In Week 11 put in 75% of your Week 1 Optimal ECPs, and in Week 12 put in 50% of your Week 1 Optimal ECPs. Week 13 is the rest week.

Table 9.2

Week	ECPs
1	
2	
3	
4	
5	
6	
7	
8	
9	
10	
11	
12	
13	0

13–Week Maintenance Program

Example:

Marlene

Week 1 ECPs = 324

Table 9.3

Week	ECPs
1	324
2	324
3	324
4	324
5	324
6	324
7	324
8	324
9	324
10	324
11	243
12	162
13	0

Marlene 13–Week Maintenance Program

PROGRESSION PROGRAM

If you decide to progress, you also will go on a 13-week program, as based upon the documented adaptation period of 10 to 12 weeks. During the first 10 weeks, your ECPs increase slightly each week. This is followed by a 2-week period of reduced ECPs that allows you to solidify adaptation or to peak for a competition or a personal challenge. As in the Maintenance Program, you take the 13th week off, which aids in the recovery of your body and keeps you fresh.

Sometimes people get concerned about taking time off. Athletes are often too hard on themselves. They don't take the time to reflect on the successes they have had and on what they have accomplished. Taking time off at the right time will help insure a lifetime of physical activity. Take the week to look back in pride and enjoy the fruits of your labor.

In the Progression Program, people with different ECPs make different progress. Progress is like going halfway toward a wall with each step: each step is only half as long as the step before. The higher your Week 1 Optimal ECPs, the closer you are to the wall, the less your percentage of progression will be. For example, if you have an energy conversion grade of A, you might make a 3% improvement on the Progression Program in a year. If you have an F, you might improve your ECPs by 40%. In terms of ECP improvement, if you have a grade of A and Week 1 Optimal ECPs of 2000, you would increase by 60 points in a year. If you have an F and Week 1 Optimal ECPs of 50, you would increase by 20 points in a year. You could not sustain a 40% increase if you started at 2000 ECPs, so ECPs increase on a sliding scale. The higher you start, the less percentage of increase you have.

The Table 9.4 lists the percentages of increase. You increase your ECPs twenty-one times in a year. Nine of those increases happen in the first 13-week cycle.

In the table, find your VO2Max. The column to the right of that number gives you the % Increase you will use.

Table 9.4

VO2Max	% Increase	VO2Max	%Increase	VO2Max	% Increase
72	.0018	52	.0086	32	.0138
71	.0021	51	.0088	31	.0141
70	.0023	50	.0091	30	.0143
69	.0028	49	.0093	29	.0146
68	.0031	48	.0098	28	.0148
67	.0033	47	.0101	27	.0151
66	.0036	46	.0103	26	.0153
65	.0038	45	.0106	25	.0156
64	.0043	44	.0108	24	.0158
63	.0046	43	.0111	23	.0161
62	.0048	42	.0113	22	.0163
61	.0051	41	.0116	21	.0166
60	.0053	40	.0118	20	.0168
59	.0056	39	.0121	19	.0171
58	.0061	38	.0123	18	.0173
57	.0068	37	.0126	17	.0176
56	.0073	36	.0128	16	.0178
55	.0076	35	.0131	15	.0181
54	.0078	34	.0133	14	.0183
53	.0081	33	.0136		

% Increase

Your % Increase = _____

Example:

Marlene

VO_2Max = 45

% Increase = .0106

Dick

VO_2Max = 50

% Increase = .0091

This is how you use your % Increase number to set up your progression program. Each 13-week cycle is done in the same manner, so when you have done the first cycle you have the process for all the rest.

Step 1. Your Week 1 Optimal ECPs = _____

Example:

Marlene

Week 1 Optimal ECPs = 324

Dick

Week 1 Optimal ECPs = 657

Step 2. Your % Increase = _____

Example:

Marlene

% Increase = .0106

Dick

% Increase = .0091

Step 3. Now you find how many ECPs you increase each time an increase occurs.

Your ECPs Increase = Week 1 Optimal ECPs x % Increase

Your ECPs Increase = _____ ECPs

Example:

Marlene

ECPs Increase = 324 x .0106 = 3 ECPs

Dick

ECPs Increase = 657 x .0091 = 6 ECPs

Step 4. Fill in the following table, and you will have your program for the first 13-week cycle. To get your optimal ECPs for each week, follow the simple directions below. It's a lot easier than Tax Form 1040.

Week 1: Enter your Week 1 Optimal ECPs.

Week 2: Enter the sum of your Week 1 Optimal ECPs plus your ECPs Increase.

Week 3: Enter the sum of Week 2 plus your ECPs Increase.

Weeks 4 through 10: Repeat by adding the previous week to the ECPs Increase.

Week 11: Enter the ECPs from Week 3.

Week 12: Subtract two (2) times the ECPs Increase from the Week 1 Optimal ECPs.

Week 13: A recovery week; 0 points has already been entered.

Table 9.5

Week	Cycle 1
1	
2	
3	
4	
5	
6	
7	
8	
9	
10	
11	
12	
13	0

13–Week Progression Program

Table 9.6

Week	Cycle 1
1	324
2	327
3	330
4	333
5	336
6	339
7	342
8	345
9	348
10	351
11	330
12	318
13	0

Marlene

Week 1 Optimal ECPs = 324

ECPs Increase = 3

Table 9.7

Week	Cycle 1
1	657
2	663
3	669
4	675
5	681
6	687
7	693
8	699
9	705
10	711
11	669
12	645
13	0

Dick

Week 1 Optimal ECPs = 657

ECPs Increase = 6

The following graph is a representation of Marlene's 13-week cycle. Her Week 1 Optimal ECPs were 324, and her % Increase equaled 3 ECPs.

Figure 9.8

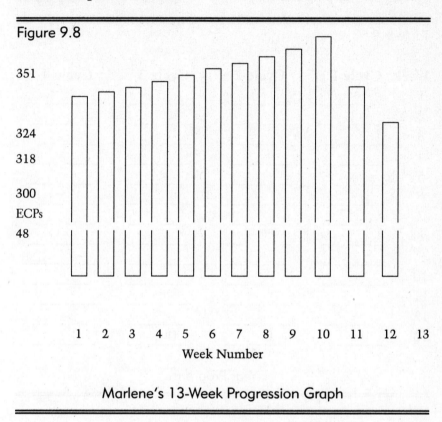

Marlene's 13-Week Progression Graph

SETTING UP A 1-YEAR PROGRAM

If you want, you can now easily set up your goals for the whole first year by blocking out four 13-week cycles. They will probably change, but determining a reasonable destination will give direction to a long-term physical activity program.

If you want a full year's Maintenance Program, all you need to do is fill in the following table by repeating the cycle for the first 13 weeks.

If you want a full year's Progression Program, repeat the instructions for Cycle 1 to fill out Cycles 2, 3, and 4. Week 1 ECPs for Cycles 2, 3, and 4 will be the optimal ECPs from Week 5 of the preceding cycle.

Table 9.9

Week	Cycle 1	Cycle 2	Cycle 3	Cycle 4
1	____	____	____	____
2	____	____	____	____
3	____	____	____	____
4	____	____	____	____
5	____	____	____	____
6	____	____	____	____
7	____	____	____	____
8	____	____	____	____
9	____	____	____	____
10	____	____	____	____
11	____	____	____	____
12	____	____	____	____
13	0	0	0	0

1-Year Program

Example:

Marlene

Table 9.10

Week	Cycle 1	Cycle 2	Cycle 3	Cycle 4
1	324	336*	348	360
2	327	339	351	363
3	330	342	354	366
4	333	345	357	369
5	336	348	360	372
6	339	351	363	375
7	342	354	366	378
8	345	357	369	381
9	348	360	372	384
10	351	363	375	387
11	330	342	354	366
12	318	330	342	354
13	0	0	0	0

*Notice that the Week 1 ECPs for the next cycle are the same as the optimal ECPs from Week 5 of the preceding cycle, and the Week 11 ECPs are the same as in Week 3 of the same cycle, and week 12 ECPs are equal to week 1 of the same cycle minus 2 times the % increase (324 – 6 = 318).

Figure 9.11

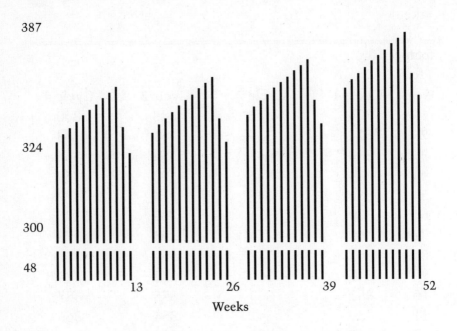

Marlene's 1-Year Progression Graph

You now have either a Maintenance or a Progression Program for a year. Neither are set in stone. There may be reasons to increase your ECPs, such as positive changes in your autobiography. You may also have to decrease them because of changes in your autobiography that reduce your ability to consume oxygen or reduce the time or support available. You can modify your ECPs whenever your autobiography changes. If you modify the ECPs, try to start the change at the beginning of a new 13-week period. Appendix B has clean copies of each table. Please copy them as often as necessary to meet the requirements of your individual L.E.A.P. program.

You might be saying, "Can't I start?" You can start anytime you want, but maybe it's worthwhile to answer a few logistical, preplanning questions. Getting the answers may take a few chapter longer, but in considering the questions you may get ideas that will help you build a better foundation and help insure that activity will become a part of your life.

CHAPTER 10

WHAT? WHEN? WHERE? PRE-PLANNING

What physical activities will you do? Where will you do them? What equipment do you need? What is the best time for you to be physically active? What clothes do you need for your physical activities? Paying attention to these questions before you start will help you get off on the right foot and be more consistent after you start.

WHAT PHYSICAL ACTIVITIES WILL YOU DO?

You should do what you enjoy doing. Choosing among fitness concepts like aerobic and anaerobic conditioning, strength training, and flexibility should come second. First, find out what you like to do, and do that. If you make physical activity an enjoyable part of your life, everything else will follow.

I was in a weight room a few months ago when I overheard someone say, "Isn't this fun?" By his emphasis and expression I knew he was being sarcastic. I felt a little sorry for him because I had learned that being physically active can be fun. Maybe it's not always fun to do some of the physical activities at a high level of intensity or to repeat some movement over and over again to gain an aerobic effect, but often physical activity *is* fun, especially if you are playing a game. And you can always count on the feeling of satisfaction that having completed a workout brings. The feeling you get after the last step, or lift, or stretch is over, after you know you have done it right and have allowed your body to express itself, is one of deep satisfaction and joy.

I have observed the apprehension athletes sometimes feel in approaching a particularly hard workout. But I have also observed the sincere and deep pleasure they feel when they have completed the workout. It is not the relief of "Thank God that's over!" It's the joy of accomplishment, the joy of a common experience, and on a deeper level, the joy of movement.

I have been privileged to be able to converse with Bill Bowerman, emeritus professor at the University of Oregon, co-founder of Nike, coach of thirty-two Olympians, and one of the fathers of the jogging movement. I have spoken with him over a period of 15 years. The first thing he always says to any runner I bring to meet him is, "If running is not fun for you, don't do it." I know he would say the same thing about any physical activity—if it's not fun, don't do it.

Three memorable moments in my coaching career, moments that made me feel good and that symbolize what a mentor should be able to do, had to do with enjoyment in the midst of stressful competition. In 1983 Mary Slaney had won the women's 3000 meters at the first World Championships in Track and Field in Helsinki, Finland. The next day, the day before the competition in the 1500-meter run began, we were eating lunch. You could feel the tension in the atmosphere surrounding us. Just at that time, she put down her fork and said, "This is really fun."

Nine years later, 1992, New Orleans: I'm quietly sitting on a bus next to Shelly Steely, an athlete I coach who had qualified as an Olympian in the 3000 meters two nights before. The bus was taking us to the stadium where she was going to run in the 1500 meters. I had never told Shelly the story about Mary. She turned to me and said, "This is really fun."

In 1994 in Monaco at a Grand Prix track and field competition, Suzy Hamilton had just finished a 1500-meter run in which she placed 7th. She said, "This is so much fun, I never want it to stop." This is how anyone can feel about physical activity if it is done right.

If you know what activities you enjoy, start with them. If you aren't sure, experiment with physical activities you think you might like or that are convenient for you to do. Try different ones. In the beginning, being physically active is all that matters. As time goes by you can add more structure to your program if you want. For example, a program that includes aerobic, anaerobic, strength, and flexibility components is very beneficial and effective, but if you stop being active because you try to do too much too soon, or try to do what people said you should do even if you don't like it, you will not make physical activity a part of your life.

There are many ways to convert energy via physical activity. Following is a list of some activities you could try. They are all included in the L.E.A.P. computer program (see Appendix N). If you aren't sure what to try, you should be able to find some ideas here. I'm sure this is not a complete list and that many of you will have ideas of other healthy activities. And you should go ahead and do these others because you know that you can convert any physical activity to ECPs using the L.E.A.P. equation:

$$ECPs = VO_{2Max}Wgt_{Coef} \times Duration \times I_{Coef}$$

L.E.A.P. ACTIVITY LIST
Adventure/Outdoor

Backpacking
Bungee Jumping
Diving
  Board
  Scuba
  Skin
  Sky
Fishing
  Bank

Rock Climbing
Skating
  Board
  Ice
  In-Line
Skiing
  Downhill
  Roller
  Water

Boat
Ocean
Wade
Hiking
Horseback Riding
Hunting
Mountain Biking
Parachuting

Snorkeling
Snowboarding
Snowshoeing
Surfing
Board
Body
Wind

Aerobics

Aerobics
Run-in-Water
Bottom
Deep
Slide Aerobics
Step Aerobics

Tread Water
Water Aerobics
Deep
Shallow

Combatant Sports

Boxing
Fencing
Judo

Karate
Wrestling
Other Martial Arts

Dance

Ballet
Ballroom
Contemporary

Modern
Tap

Distance/Pace Activities[1]

Bicycling
Cross-Country Skiing
Jogging or Running
Jogging and Walking
Racewalking
Swimming
Treadmill

Walking
Heavy Hands
Normal
Rapid
Wheelchair Push

---

[1]In distance/pace activities, special types of workouts, such as fartlek, interval, racing, and tempo, are implied. (These terms are defined in Appendix I.) When using RPE, the intensities involved in these activities are automatically considered. In the L.E.A.P. computer program the user has the ability to define these types of workouts more completely by using pace or distance and recovery intervals where appropriate.

Exercise Equipment/Machines

Airdyne–type Machine
Bicycle
   Recumbent Stationary
   Spinning
   Upright Stationary
Concept II–type Rowing Machine
Healthrider–type Machine
Jump Rope
Nordic Track–type Skiing Machine
Stair Climbing
Stair Master–type Machine
Trampoline
   Mini
   Regular
VersaClimber–type Machine

Games/Sports[2]

Archery
Badminton
Baseball
Basketball
Billiards
Bowling
Croquet
Football
   Tackle
   Touch
Frisbee
Golf
   Cart
   Driving Range
   Walk
Gymnastics
Handball
Hockey
   Field
   Ice
   Street

Horseshoes
Lacrosse
Paddleball
Racquetball
Rugby
Shooting
Schuffleboard
Soccer
Softball
Squash
Table Tennis
Tennis
   Singles
   Doubles
Volleyball
   Court
   Sand
Wallyball

---

[2]Games or sports often involve drills or just practicing the prime task, like shooting in basketball.

Home/Work Activities

Bed Rehabilitation Exercises
Gardening
Housework

Manual Labor
Rehabilitation Exercises
Sexual Activity

Strength/Flexibility Training

Body Building
Calisthenics
Circuit Training
Stretching

Weight Training
  Endurance
  Power
  Strength
  Tone
Yoga

Water Craft

Canoeing
Jet Boating
Kayaking
Rafting
Rowing
  Boat
  Shell

Sail Boarding
Sailing
  Lake
  Ocean

In selecting activities, you will have to consider whether some of the negatives about some activities will eventually cause you to stop doing them. Some can be done only at a specific time. Others are restricted to what an exercise leader might want you to do. Some activities may be difficult to access or pose physical danger. Certain activities may be boring or may restrict you to one location.

On the other hand, some of these same activities may provide you with physical and psychological benefits. Others will provide support groups. Some can be done almost anyplace and anytime. Some are part of a normal day and others are done in pristine, beautiful settings. Some will generate a passion. Those that are exciting, enjoyable, and fun will enhance the probability that you will remain active.

Personal choice is extremely important. A key to a good start is choosing not activities you feel you *need* to do but activities you feel you would *like* to do. Start with activities that you believe will be enjoyable.

DOES THE ACTIVITY REQUIRE EQUIPMENT?

"I'm going to start being physically active. I better go out and buy a _____." You all know of friends who have some exercise equipment sitting in their garage. They probably said the same thing. Depending upon what you want to do, you may need some equipment. But as you have seen from the L.E.A.P. Activity List, it's certainly not necessary to go out and buy expensive equipment. Here are my basic thoughts on equipment.

SHOES

Other than your body, the most important piece of equipment you will use is a good pair of shoes. Most physical activities take place against gravity with the feet touching the ground. Sometimes they touch the ground many times in a short period. Each time the foot hits the ground, the impact is many times greater than body weight. The forces of impact reverberate not only in the lower extremities but throughout the body, which is why the purpose of good footwear is to solve the problems that arise when the foot strikes and leaves the ground.

Basically there are two major considerations: absorption of forces and alignment of body parts. Correct shoes moderate both considerations, protecting the weight-bearing bones and joints of the body and, through injury-free training, aiding performance.

What shoes should you buy? There is no single correct answer. There are different shoes for different activities and occasionally even different shoes for different aspects of the same activity. More important, while there is no perfect shoe for everyone, there is a correct shoe for you.

Your foot type is the major factor that dictates what basic shoe type you should consider. There are two basic foot types: (1) high-arched and fairly rigid and (2) low-arched, fairly flat, and flexible. Although it's best to have a professional analyze your feet if you have problems, you can do a quick check to get a general idea. After you take a shower look at your footprints. If the print looks like two balls connected by a narrow strip, you probably have high-arched, fairly rigid feet. If the print looks more like a rectangle, you probably have low-arched and fairly flat feet. The rigid foot seems to do better in shoes that are flexible and have cushioning. The flat foot seems to do better in shoes that are more firm and stable.

Knowing the parts of an athletic shoe can help you understand what to look for when you shop for the shoe that will suit your needs best. There are five basic parts of a shoe: outer sole, midsole, last, upper, and heel counter.

Starting from the bottom up, the *outer sole* is the part that has contact with the ground. Traction is an important aspect of the outer sole, as is durability. Often, depending upon footstrike, parts of the shoe may wear at different rates. Some shoes are made with a nonuniform outer sole to compensate for uneven wear. For example, the outer edge of the heel often wears more rapidly, so there may be more durable material in this area. As durability increases so does weight, which at some point becomes a disadvantage. So there may be a cost/benefit ratio to take into account when you make your buying decision.

The *midsole* lies on top of the outer sole. It is the primary shock absorber when the foot lands, and its most important feature is how much it will compact and then spring back to its original thickness. The softer it is, the more shock it will absorb and the more you can indent it with your thumb. The harder it is, the less shock it will absorb and the less you can indent it with your thumb. Even though it may seem that softer is better, there is a trade-off for a low-arched foot. The midsole must be hard enough to resist inward rotation, which happens to a greater extent with a low-arched foot, as the foot progresses from landing to toe-off. The midsole must also be flexible enough to bend under the forefoot as the heel comes off the ground. Sometimes nonuniform midsoles are part of the shoe. The heel, the inside half of the shoe (from the back to the middle of the foot), and across the shoe under the forefoot are often made of different materials to improve pronation resistance and flexibility.

The *last*, from the Old English for *footprint*, is the pattern from which the shoe is made. There are straight-lasted and curve-lasted shoes. On the bottom of a straight-lasted shoe you can draw a straight line from the middle of the back of the shoe to the middle of the front of the shoe. This type of last counteracts pronation and provides additional support for low-arched feet. On the bottom of a curve-lasted shoe the line from back to front curves inward. This type of last enhances absorption and flexibility and works better for someone who has high-arched feet.

The *upper* is the part of the shoe that attaches to the midsole and covers the top of the foot. It is usually made of nylon because this material is light, resists shrinkage, and dries quickly. You may hear the terms *slip-lasting* and *board-lasting*. Slip-lasting means that there is nothing between the foot and the point of contact between the upper of the shoe and the midsole. This enhances flexibility and is better for high-arched feet. Board-lasting means that there is a full board, running the length of the shoe, or a partial board, running half the length of the shoe, between the foot and where the upper of the shoe attaches to the midsole. This improves stability in the shoe and provides more support for the low-arched foot.

The *heel counter* is not always needed. Often people prefer to modify the top of the heel counter because it can be irritating as opposed to helpful. However, it is a support structure built at the heel of the shoe to help reduce ankle pronation. If you have low-arched feet, you should consider a shoe with a firm heel counter.

These are not all the features shoes may have, but they are basic to all designs. Couple this technical information with the advertising and the numerous and constantly changing models, and buying a pair of shoes can become intimidating. There are hundreds of models from which to choose. How do you choose the right pair of shoes for you?

First, buy from an athletic shoe speciality store. Shoe companies often send representatives to these stores to educate the employees on the features of the models they carry. These employees are generally interested in physical activity and can help identify the type of foot you have. They understand that the type of physical activity, the surfaces, and the frequency of activity all help determine what type of shoe you need.

It isn't necessary to get the most expensive shoe. That doesn't always equate to the most effective one. You should start by looking at a minimal shoe, the cheapest, lightest one you can safely use. These can often be purchased for between $50 and $70.

It is also beneficial to try on many different models. When you try on a shoe, if it doesn't feel good immediately, don't buy it in the hope that you will "break it in." If it doesn't feel good right away, it's not for you.

The size of the shoes should be about a half size bigger than you normally take. This is due to the swelling of the feet that sometimes occurs during activity. A good guideline, suggested by Dr. Tim Nokes, is what he calls the "index finger test." There should be a space the width of your index finger between the end of your longest toe and the end of the shoe. The width and height of the front part of the shoe should also allow for freedom of movement of the toes. Finally, your foot should not slip out of the heel counter as you lift the foot off the ground when you run or walk.

Once you have found a shoe you really like, it is a good idea to buy extra pairs. The way shoe models change like new cars each year, it is worth having a reserve in order to rotate shoes and to insure that you always have shoes that work.

Shoes do wear out, and it is better to buy a new pair than to try to repair the old ones, even if it looks as if you made a successful repair. The resiliency of the midsole is something you can't repair, and this property declines with age, so it is always better to replace shoes sooner rather than later.

You might be interested in an all-purpose athletic shoe. This is a good choice when you are beginning your physical activity program. Because these shoes combine shock absorption with lateral stability, they can be used for a number of different activities. It should be remembered that they are a compromise, and if you want to specialize in an activity you should consider shoes made specifically for that activity.

EQUIPMENT

If you want to buy exercise equipment, first consider that you can probably join a good health club for several years for what you may pay for appropriate equipment. But if you want to have some equipment at your private disposal at home, try it several times before you purchase it. Probably before you even try it you can find out a lot about it by going to several athletic equipment stores and getting their opinions, prices, and brochures. You can also go to health clubs and ask about what brand of equipment they purchase and why. They are often helpful, especially if you go to a locally owned club. Many will allow you to try their equipment for one or more times. And often you can take advantage of the fact that many clubs will give you a free trial membership for a few days or a week with the hope you will become a member.

If your physical activity calls for equipment that you want to purchase, buying it can be an enjoyable experience but should not be taken lightly. The equipment is something that you hope will become a part of your life. With respect to length and quality of life, it may be more important than the purchase of a car. Just as with any purchase, there are levels of quality. Look for durability, reliability, and some accurate way to measure what you are doing. Forget readouts of calories because the machine doesn't know you as an individual. What you want is some way to accurately measure distance and time, or pace and time. Some equipment will give you the choice of doing a variety of workouts. As long as you get to know these workouts slowly and don't go for the harder levels at first, these suggestions provide some early guidance.

HEART RATE MONITORS

A heart rate monitor can be a valuable piece of equipment because it can provide accurate information about intensity. It is not crucial to making physical activity a part of your life, but if you enjoy accurate feedback you could consider a good heart rate monitor. If you are going to invest in one, make sure you buy one with a chest strap that sends the signal to a monitor worn like a wristwatch. Picking up the pulse from the wrist only, with no chest leads, is either not as reliable or more expensive.

To use a heart rate monitor most effectively you should know your accurate resting and maximum heart rates so you can determine your heart rate reserve. The heart rate reserve is the maximum heart rate minus the resting heart rate. Maximum heart rate should be determined by a stress test under the supervision of qualified person. Using formulas adjusted for age is not an accurate method for determining maximum heart rate. Another advantage of a well-conducted stress test is that it will indicate where your lactate production exceeds your lactate removal. Knowing the approximate heart rate at which this occurs allows you to stay in your steady state zone.

Another reason a heart rate monitor may be useful is that it can alert you to overtraining. For example, if a run of 2 miles that you've been doing in 16 minutes requires a higher heart rate to do under the same environmental conditions, you know your body has not recovered from the last workout. Conversely, if your heart rate is lower for the same workout, you know your body is adapting.

See Appendix D for more about heart rate.

WHERE WILL YOU BE ACTIVE?

There are two qualities the place you are active should have. First, you should like being there. Second, it should "take you away."

The place can be indoors or out. It can be a club or your own home. It can be a court or a field. It can be somewhere to play a game with a lot of friends and competitors or somewhere you can be alone or with a special friend. The place can be several places, depending upon what you want to do.

Wherever your place for physical activity is, you should look forward to going there and being there. As you are going, you should feel a subtle anticipation because you know you like being at that place. When you arrive, you should feel some sense of detachment from the rest of your life. If it is a health club or YMCA, you should enjoy interacting with the employees and the other members, even if it is just a friendly exchange of hellos. You should feel you belong. The physical atmosphere of the place should give you pleasure. If you are using equipment, the place should have equipment you enjoy using.

The place should also take you away from your work and responsibilities. There should be no phone to interrupt your physical activity, your mental concentration on the enjoyment of the physical activity, and the drift away from other cares. Business and personal situations should take a backseat while you are being active. Others seeking to intrude on your island of tranquility should know enough to respect its boundaries and to continue the intrusion only if it is clear you welcome it. Your place for physical activity should be "your place." And you should be able to say, "I really like being here."

WHEN WILL YOU BE ACTIVE?

Two factors determine when you should be active. First, physical activity should coincide with the flow of your circadian rhythms. This automatically happens if you do the physical activity at the same time of day, at a time you know is a good part of the day for you. If you do the activity at a time when you are not usually active or that you know is not your time of day, you will probably be out of sync with your circadian rhythm Second, physical activity should have a place on your schedule, so you know it is a planned part of your day.

The productivity of people varies. Some are very effective in the early morning. Some do their best work at night. The same is true with physical activity. Some people thrive, or have learned to thrive, on doing their physical activity in the morning soon after they wake up. Others look forward to getting in their workout after their workday in the late afternoon or early evening. Still others look forward to being physically active in the middle of the day; it seems to set them up for a more productive afternoon. Some have become adept at making use of scraps of time and fitting in the activity when their schedule permits.

Nobody can tell you when you should be active. You are the best person to determine that. You know what works best for you. When you have determined that time, the attitude you should take is that it is as important as any other obligation on your schedule. It is an obligation to yourself.

WHAT CLOTHING IS BEST
SUITED FOR YOUR ACTIVITY?

As with equipment, if you require special clothing, such as a helmet or wet suit or gloves, you are well advised to get the best quality even if the cost seems somewhat high. Where safety is concerned you must look at clothing as insurance. The right clothing will insure your maximum enjoyment.

However, unless your activity requires special clothing for safety or performance, there is no reason to be a fashion plate. Comfortable clothing that wicks moisture away from the body is all you need in a warm environment. Several layers of comfortable clothing is all you need in a cool or cold environment.

This is what I mean. Suppose it is a warm day. You are best off with a light-colored natural fiber, probably cotton. Being light colored, it will reflect heat. Dark colors absorb heat, making it harder for your body to maintain temperature homeostasis, which makes your body work harder to stay cool. On a hot day, out in the sun, put your hand on something colored white and something colored black. You can feel the difference color makes. On a warm day when you are working out, the temperature in your body rises because you produce heat when your muscles contract. The blood must carry the heat away from the vital organs to the skin. At the skin the heat is then carried out of the body in sweat. If the sweat evaporates, you enhance the cooling effect.

Cotton wicks moisture away from the body, where it can evaporate in the air instead of rolling off your body. To make something go from a liquid (water, sweat), which is cooler, to a gas (water vapor), which is hotter, requires energy. The heat in the water vapor is removed from the proximity of your body when the water evaporates, which produces the cooling effect. Synthetic fabrics and blends do not wick as well as cotton unless they are specially designed to do so, in which case they are more expensive.

Clothing that fits tightly doesn't wick as well as loose-fitting clothing and often restricts movement in addition to enhancing irritation. Clothing with a lot of printing on it doesn't wick as well either.

If you do your physical activity outdoors on cold days, you should wear layers of clothing that wick and protect key areas of the body. You want to keep your body warm, so the blood is not shunted away from the muscles to warm the core. Your fingers and toes can get cold and your limbs can get cold, but if your core temperature drops just a few degrees you are in trouble. If you have inadequate clothing, this shunting will occur, reducing the blood to your muscles.

By wearing layers of light, fairly loose-fitting clothing that wick, you are accomplishing two important goals. First, the layers will trap air between them, and this air will retain some of your body heat, creating a layer of insulation between your skin and the environment. It is much like the hair of an animal that rises in cold weather, entrapping an insulating layer of air. We still have the remnants of this physiological function in goose bumps. If we had more hair, these would act to raise that hair and trap the air.

Second, on cold days the wicking keeps the skin dryer, which is an advantage because the more moisture next to the skin on cold days, the cooler the skin. Also, when you stop your activity, the more moisture you have next to your skin the faster you cool down. This is a situation that can enhance your risk of developing a cold or flu because it affects immune system function. Wool is another natural fiber that wicks very well and is warmer than cotton.

There are several areas of the body that require more protection on cold days. You want to protect your head because almost 25% of the heat lost is lost through the scalp. You want to protect the throat and upper respiratory area because you want to make the air going to the lungs as warm as possible. As air passes through the throat and bronchial areas it is warmed. If those areas are not protected, the air is not as warm as it could be when it enters the lungs and therefore the exchange of oxygen is not as efficient. In addition, the enzymes and immune system molecules that help filter and fight invaders don't function as well in cold air and you are at greater risk of picking up an upper respiratory tract infection. You also want to protect your fingers because if you can keep them artificially warm via clothing, not as much blood needs to be shunted to them, and it can be used in the muscles for physical activity.

There is nothing quite like a brisk workout on a cold day to make you feel a part of nature. Which in reality we are, even though our culture and the technology it has produced seek to remove us from the fluctuations of the natural world. When you go out-of-doors on a cold day to be physically active, this is what I think you should wear. Actually it's what I always wore when I ran in the middle of a winter day in Maine. Some days it was 20 below with a wind-chill added on. As it got warmer I could wear less and less.

Head   Wool Ski Mask—covered head, ears, and cheeks
       (breathed through wool over mouth to warm the air)
Neck   Wool Turtleneck Dickey
       (warmed throat and upper chest area)
Chest Cotton T-Shirt (then the dickey)
       Long-Sleeved Wool T-Shirt
       Cotton T-Shirt
       Cheap, Light, Insulated Hunting Vest
       Moderate-Weight Wool Sweatshirt
Hands Cotton Sweat Socks
       (all five fingers together help warm each other)
Legs   Light-Weight Wool Long Underwear Pants
       Cotton Sweat Pants
Feet   Cotton Sweat Socks
       Running Shoes

I may not have looked stylish, but the clothing was comfortably loose and light, and I was pleasantly warm. Invariably, even on the coldest day, I ended up carrying the socks I used for my hands because my hands were so warm.

Whatever you wear, safety is first, evaporation or insulation is second, efficiency and comfort are third. Style need not count.

A final thought about clothing. I have found that if you have a place where your clean workout clothes wait, it makes it easier to get out the door and be active. It seems like such a small thing, but it makes a significant difference at the time when the activity commitment is to be fulfilled. If you have to run around and gather your clothing—a T-shirt here, a towel there, your shoes in another place, your shorts in the dryer—it just gives you one more subconscious reason not to do the physical activity that day. If you know that all your workout clothing is in your gym bag by the door, it makes it easier for you to get out the door. Having a place where your clean clothes wait is a small but effective trick on your mind that helps you make physical activity a part of your life.

Once you have a good pair of shoes, the equipment your activity might require, a place to be active, and the right clothes, you're just about ready to begin. I just need to tell you about the advantages of keeping a record of your physical activity.

CHAPTER 11

THE L.E.A.P. LOGS

A key part of the L.E.A.P. program is keeping a log. A log is satisfying to fill in, important to have, and enjoyable to review. Once you've done the physical work, not recording it won't take it away from your body. But recording it in a log makes physical activity more a part of your life.

First, to make L.E.A.P. most effective it helps to track your daily ECPs and see how you're progressing toward your weekly goal.

Second, it helps to verify that the physical activity you just did was something of value when you take the time to write it down. It is satisfying to see in black and white that you did something for yourself. The immediate feedback enhances your sense of achievement.

Third, having a written record constantly encourages you. You look back and realize what you've done. You feel good about yourself. The positive feedback acts as a stimulus to help you keep physical activity a part of your life.

Fourth, comparing what you did with what you are doing is an easy way to verify progress or be alerted to problem areas. If you do a particular workout several times over a period of 4 or 5 weeks, and after each workout your leg hurts, by having recorded that information you may be able to pick up the connection between activity and pain before a more serious injury occurs. Or you may see that you thrive on a certain workout and be more inclined to duplicate it. Or maybe you jogged a particular route in 15 minutes, and now you are covering the same distance in 14 minutes. Once again you feel good about yourself and are reinforced in your desire to make physical activity a part of your life.

Fifth, your log shows you where you are going. You set out a destination or goal. Are you reaching that goal? The log is part of your road map. You can see where you have been, where you are, and where you are heading.

Recording your physical activity in a log is an efficient investment of time. It probably takes no more than a minute to record what you did. Where it takes time is when you sit and look back through it feeling good about yourself. But you don't mind taking that time. I have often seen people just sit and page through their activity diary, enjoying every minute of their reflections and drawing energy and information from those reflections.

YOUR L.E.A.P. WEEKLY LOG

Your log can be as simple or as complex as you want. A sample log is shown in Table 11.1. Across the top there is space for you to write your $VO_2MaxWgt_{Coef}$ so you don't have to multiply by VO_2Max and weight and then divide by 1936. Also across the top are spaces for the beginning of the success, optimal, and overtraining zones, the four levels, and 40% of your weekly ECPs so that you can write them in and be reminded of their values.

The next row has a heading for Days, and the days are numbered so that you can make any day the start of your week. Then there is a space for the activities you do. Record as many activities as you do each day. Remember, your activity choices are extensive and are essentially limited only by your imagination. Duration, in minutes, and I_{Coef} are the next two columns. Following are four columns, one for the ECPs earned for each activity, one for the total ECPs earned that day, one for the weekly running total of ECPs, and one for the ECPs remaining in the week. This last column can be very valuable, not only so

Table 11.1

Date _____ $VO_{2}Max$ _____ Success Zone ≥ _____ Optimal Zone ≥ Optimal Level = Overtng Zone> 40% ECPs = _____ Risk Reduction = _____
Cycle _____ WgtCoef= _____ Body Change = _____
Week _____ $VO_{2}MaxChange$ = _____

Day	Activities	Duration (min)	ICoef	ECPs (Act)	Total ECPs (day)	Total (wk)	ECPs Left	Comments
1								
2								
3								
4								
5								
6								
7								
Totals		Total Time	ECPs/Min			Total ECPs		Zone (Circle 1)

Success/Optimal/OT

Sample L.E.A.P. Weekly Log

that you can see how you are progressing, but also because it gives you a number you can use to determine exactly how much more you have to do each week to reach your goal.

Let's say the ECPs Remaining column showed that you had 50 ECPs left to reach your goal for the week. You could manipulate Duration and Intensity to figure out exactly how much more activity you should do to accomplish what was exactly right for you that week.

In the Comments section you can write what was unique about the activity, the environment, or your physical and mental reactions. Often the Comments section, on review, turns out to provide important clues that help keep physical activity a part of your life.

Across the bottom you can total the time you spent being physically active during the week. You can also total your ECPs and see how close you came to your goal. There is a place for you to circle which zone you attained. There is also a space for ECPs per minute. This is a measure of your average intensity for the week, and it is obtained by dividing ECPs by Duration. For example, if Marlene scored 339 ECPs for the week and was active for 570 minutes, her average intensity would be .60 ECPs/min. From the intensity scale, this means her average workout was done at an intensity of approximately 58% VO2Max. Over time it is interesting and instructive to observe how intensity varies from week to week.

THE L.E.A.P. 13-WEEK LOG

The L.E.A.P. 13-Week Log can serve as a progress-at-a-glance summary sheet. On it you can record the duration, total ECPs for the week, and average ECPs/min. You can also make a check mark in the appropriate level and zone to see at a glance how well you did that week.

If you would like to estimate the number of *calories you converted* each week, all you need to do is to multiply ECPs

Table 11.2

Cycle	Duration	ECPs	ECPs/Min	Success Zone	Optimal Zone	Overtng Zone	Calories= (ECPs x 4.85)	Pounds Not Gained= (Cal÷3500)
1								
2								
3								
4								
5								
6								
7								
8								
9								
10								
11								
12								
13								
Totals								

Sample L.E.A.P. 13-Week Log

by 4.85. Remember, ECPs are the same as liters of oxygen consumed, and for each liter of oxygen consumed, between 4.2 and 5 calories are converted. This method provides an estimate, or ballpark figure, of caloric conversion. You can take the idea of caloric conversion a step further and figure out how how many *pounds you did not gain* because you were active. No one can say you will lose weight when you are active, because there are other factors, such as diet, that contribute to weight gain or loss. But what can be said is that because you were active, you did not gain X number of pounds over a period of time. To figure this out, just divide the number of calories by 3500, the number of calories in 1 pound of fat.

The number of pounds you did not gain each week may seem small, and you may say, "Why bother?" Here's why. Even if Marlene only reached her risk reduction level of 126 ECPs, she would convert 611 calories. That means she did not gain .18 pounds that week, because she was physically active. Now if she is active 48 of the 52 weeks at just the risk reduction level, she will have not gained *8.4 pounds*. She will weigh almost 9 pounds less than she would have if she had done no physical activity. Maybe even that doesn't seem like much. But remember that (1) she was active at only the risk reduction level, (2) we have not even discussed the effects of diet, and (3) lifetime physical activity is a long-term process.

Now look 5 years down the road. You can see that because Marlene was physically active at just the risk reduction level, she weighs 42 pounds less than she would if she had not been active. Now it's starting to mean something.

Obviously, you can't continue this line of thinking until you waste away to nothing. There will be a point where your body hits a level of body weight that is the right weight for you. Then you will eat enough to maintain that weight, and physical activity will keep you healthy at that weight.

The weekly log and the 13-week log give you the ability to see exactly where you are in your training program. You immediately see when you have not done enough, when you have done what is right for you, and when you have done too much. Since you are getting constant feedback, it is much harder to get lost.

PART 3

FINE-TUNING

You now have two powerful numbers: your Energy Conversion Number, from which you determined your Energy Conversion Points (ECPs). These numbers enable you to start the L.E.A.P. program at a place that is right for you, to develop an ongoing program, and to measure your success as you participate in the program.

This section will show you how to use the ECPs by taking you through a sample week. And then I'll try to anticipate questions you may have when different situations arise as you try to make physical activity a part of your life.

CHAPTER 12

GOING THROUGH A SAMPLE WEEK

So far I have used Marlene and myself as examples. Now, as a change of pace, I'll use a recent week from one of the athletes I coach. Her name is Vicki Huber, and she has had the good fortune to have been on two Olympic teams. In the 1988 Summer Olympic Games in Seoul, Korea, while being coached by Marty Sterns of Villanova, where she went to college, she was a finalist in the women's 3000-meter run. Then, 13 months after the birth of her daughter, Alyssa, she made the 1996 Olympic team in the women's 1500-meter run at the Atlanta games. She is now training for the year 2000 games in Sydney.

This example uses Vicki's 8th week from Cycle 1 of a progression program. At that time Vicki's numbers were:

Energy Conversion Number = 21.73
VO_2Max = 57 ml/kg/min

This correlates nicely with predictions from the Daniels Oxygen Power Performance Tables. In these tables Dr. Daniels accurately correlates VO_2Max with running times. These estimate her VO_2Max to be near 58.6 ml/kg/min based on a recent 5-km run in 17:23 minutes.

Week 1 ECPs	= 1374	
% Increase	= .0068	= 9 ECPs
Optimal ECPs Goal for Week 8	= 1437	

Vicki's levels and zones for Week 8 are shown below.

Table 12.1

	≥148 **Success Zone**	≥1329 **Optimal Zone**	≥1545 **Overtraining Zone**
Safe	Risk Reduction = 148	Optimal = 1437	
Minimum	Body Change = 188		
	VO2Max Change = 251		

Levels and Zones Vicki Huber Week 8

Vicki has a planned weekly training schedule that at this time of the year is divided into four parts:

1. A major training run each day divided into percentage of total weekly running time for the major runs each day (we train on time and effort, not on miles)
2. An easy recovery effort,[1] running or bike or water, each day except Sunday
3. Strides or easy speed[2] incorporated into the major training run on two out of three possible days each week, or a tempo run/race[3] substituted for speed/strides on Saturday
4. Weight training two out of three possible days a week

---

[1]Recovery effort: an easy physical activity of short duration and low intensity whose goal is to enhance recovery by promoting increased circulation without stimulating a real physical challenge.

[2]Strides/easy speed: a pickup in speed that lasts for 50 to 100 meters during part of a longer run. It may be repeated 5 to 10 times during the run. Technique and turnover are the goals.

[3]Tempo run: a run in which you are challenged but in control. You should be able to start and finish at the same pace. When the run is complete, you should feel tired but exhilarated, not exhausted.

Table 12.2 displays Vicki's suggested training schedule with the approximate goal ECPs for each workout. You will notice that her actual log follows the pattern but is not an exact replica. Guidelines are not mandates. We rarely do a workout exactly as planned. They are modified according to an athlete's needs and environmental conditions.

Table 12.2

Day	Major train-ing run	Recovery Effort	Strides/Speed Tempo/Race	Weight Training	Est. ECPs/day
Sunday	22%				264
Monday	10%	x			150
Tuesday	15%	x	Strides/Speed	x	240
Wednesday	10%	x			150
Thursday	18%	x	Strides/Speed	x	276
Friday	10%	x			150
Saturday	15%	x	Tempo/Race	x	210
				Total	1440

Suggested Training Schedule for Vicki Huber

Day 1—On Sunday Vicki ran 84 minutes at an intensity of approximately 75% VO2Max. To do this she consumed 193 liters of oxygen and earned 193 ECPs.

ECPs = 1.91 x 84 x 1.20 = 193

Day 2—On Monday Vicki did a morning recovery workout in the water and then a 45-minute run. These are her calculations for the two workouts.

ECPs A.M. = 1.91 x 20 x .51 = 20
ECPs P.M. = 1.91 x 45 x 1.40 = 120

Day 3—On Tuesday she decided that this would be one of her weight training days. She does weights after her major run. By doing the weights after her major run she converts energy at a higher rate for a longer period of time, and by doing it on the days of a harder running workout her easy days are easier and provide for more recovery. On this Tuesday Vicki did a 10-minute recovery run, a 65-minute run at 85% VO2Max, and 40 minutes of weight training.

ECPs A.M. = 1.91 x 10 x .51 = 10
ECPs P.M. = 1.91 x 65 x 1.62 = 201
ECPs Weights = 1.91 x 40 x .66 = 50

Day 4—On Wednesday, just to be safe Vicki went into the water again. I encourage athletes to use deep water cross-training anytime they want, even if they feel great. Your joints get to recover and you can always get a good cardiovascular workout in the water. In the afternoon she did the 45 minutes but ran at an easy pace. Athletes know that they have a range of paces they can choose to run depending upon how they feel. The pace range correlates with a 70% to 85% VO2Max.

ECPs A.M. = 1.91 x 20 x .16 = 6
ECPs P.M. = 1.91 x 45 x 1.00 = 86

Day 5—On Thursday Vicki sees that she is approaching her optimal goal but knows that she can adjust on a easy day, so she decides to do the workout scheduled and chooses this day as her second weight day. She does back off a little on the recovery run because she knows that recovery runs can be between 10 and 20 minutes.

ECPs A.M. = 1.91 x 10 x .51 = 10
ECPs P.M. = 1.91 x 75 x 1.86 = 266
ECPs Weights = 1.91 x 35 x .82 = 55

Day 6—On Friday Vicki knows that to reach her optimal ECPs she has only 420 points remaining. But she is feeling good and still wants to do the tempo run planned on Saturday, so she has to play a what-if game to see how she can schedule the rest of her week. She decides that unless something changes she will try to be near optimal level, which is 1437 ECPs.

She knows the tempo run is planned to be 5 km and that she hopes to run it in about 17:00. She knows the effort will be close to 90% VO2Max. But she also knows that she will have a warm-up and a warm-down, which at this time of year will be part warm-down and part training run. Then she'll have the recovery run later in the afternoon. So now she sees how many ECPs will accumulate on Saturday if things go according to plan. I'll use italics to show that this is a what-if planning exercise.

ECPs Warm-Up = 1.91 x 15 x 1.00 = 29
ECPs Tempo = 1.91 x 17 x 2.10 = 68
ECPs Warm-Down = 1.91 x 40 x 1.62 = 123
ECPs Recovery Run = 1.91 x 20 x .51 = 20

Her projected total for Saturday appears to be 240 ECPs, which gives her about 180 (420 - 240) ECPs to work with on Friday. So it looks as if she'll have no trouble staying near her optimal level.

Doing the math is easy and in no way takes away from the enjoyment and challenge of training. In fact, it makes it more enjoyable because Vicki knows she will be doing what is right for her.

On Friday she does her morning recovery run and then has the training run in the afternoon as planned.

ECPs A.M. = 1.91 x 20 x .51 = 20
ECPs P.M. = 1.91 x 48 x 1.4 = 128

Day 7—On Saturday she does the tempo as planned and feels better at the faster pace and a little harder intensity than she thought she would. Her time is 16:52.

ECPs Warm-Up = 1.91 x 25 x 1.00 = 48
ECPs Tempo = 1.91 x 16.87 x 2.63 = 85
ECPs Warm-Down = 1.91 x 35 x 1.40 = 94
ECPs Recovery Run = 1.91 x 20 x .51 = 20

At the end of the week Vicki was in her ECPs optimal zone, near her optimal level, so it all turned out fine. She met her training goals and had a good tempo effort. She doesn't have to worry about what other athletes are doing. She knows that she is doing what is best for her.

Table 12.3

Date 10/5 Cycle 1 Week 8	VO2Max WgtCoef= 1.91	Success Zone≥ 1519	Optimal Zone≥ 1329	Optimal Level≥ 1437	Overtng Zone> 608	40% ECPs 575		Risk Red=148 Body Chg=188 VO2Change=251
Day	Activities	Duration (min)	ICoef	ECPs (Act)	Total (day)	Total (week)	ECPs Left	Comments
1	Run	84	1.20	193	193	193	1244	Clare, Marla Jen, and Guy
2	Water	20	0.51	20	140	333	1104	Felt a little
	Run	45	1.40	120				tired this am
3	Run	10	0.51	10	261	594	843	Knee felt
	Run	65	1.62	201				best it has
	Weights	40	0.66	50				
4	Water	20	0.16	6	92	686	751	Felt good to
	Run	45	1.00	86				take it easy
5	Run	10	0.51	10	331	1027	410	Hard run
	Run	75	1.86	266				with some
	Weights	35	0.82	55				hills
6	Run	20	0.51	20	148	1165	272	Might feel a
	Run	48	1.40	128				little tired for
								tempo, but easy
7	Warm-up	25	1.00	48	247	1412	25	Really good
	Tempo	16.87	2.63	85				tempo felt
	Warm-dwn	35	1.40	94				under control
	Run	20	0.51	20				
	Total Time		ECPs/Min			Total ECPs		ZONE (Circle 1)
Totals		613.87	2.30			1412		Success/*Optimal*/OT

Weely Log for Vicki Huber—Week 8

As athletes go through the week, questions always come up, just as they do for any of us. In the next chapter I try to anticipate some of the more common ones.

CHAPTER 13

FREQUENTLY ASKED QUESTIONS

You now know the basic rules of L.E.A.P. and have the tools to make the program work for you, but there are several forks in the road in the form of questions or situations that can arise. Having the answers to these questions beforehand, or knowing where to find the answers when they arise, will help you be more successful with L.E.A.P. I call these answers fine-tuning and pose the questions in the form of "What if. . . ?"

First, another example of the best case, reaching your optimal zone, in the form of a 1-week log from Marlene.

Table 12.3

Date 9/7 Cycle 1 Week 1	VO2Max WgtCoef= 1.58	Success Zone≥ 123	Optimal Zone≥ 300	Optimal Level= 324	Overtng Zone> 348	40% ECPs 130			Risk Red=123 Body Chg=156 VO2Change=207
Day	Activities	Duration (min)	ICoef	ECPs (Act)	Total (day)	Total (week)	ECPs Left		Comments
1	Housework	60	0.51	48	48	48	276		Should have done more
2	Office Walking	90	0.26	37	37	85	239		
3	Office Walking	80	0.26	33	33	118	206		
4	Office Walking Walk to Bank	80 30	0.26 0.51	33 25	58	176	148		
5	Office Walking	70	.37	41	41	217	107		Very busy at office
6	Office Walking Walk at Lunch	55 30	.26 .82	23 39	62	279	45		Great early fall day
7	Gardening	75	.51	60	60	339	-15		Nice day to be outside
		Total Time	ECPs/Min			Total ECPs			ZONE (Circle 1)
		570	0.60			339			Success/*Optimal*/OT

Marlene Weekly Log—Week 1

Marlene reached her optimal zone. You can also see that she made an estimate of the total time she spent walking and doing various physical tasks at her job in the doctor's office. On the 4th and 6th days she did two activities and recorded both of them. She stayed well under her 40% level of energy conversion per day. She also made some comments. Not all comments are germane, but over time comments form a pattern and will give you clues to your ability to convert energy.

Summing up at the end of the week gives you the week at a glance. The ECPs per minute are interesting because they represent a summary of the average intensity of your physical activities.

Marlene estimated her intensity, for each activity. *Estimating* is the key concept when dealing with intensity. As long as you try to be honest with yourself, you will always get a consistent measurement of your intensity.

I've had questions like "What if I lift weights, do I estimate the intensity as I am doing the lifting or when I finish?" Estimating intensity on intermittent activities like weight lifting is done after you finish. You think about things like how long you lifted, how hard it felt, how long you rested between the lifts, and how much recovery you felt you had. You have clues to work with like how hard you were breathing and how well you could talk. Maybe the %VO2Max you come up with won't be bulls-eye accurate. But if you are honest you will be relatively accurate, and the ECPs will reflect a consistent measurement of your energy conversion in that activity. If you are true to yourself, you won't be trying to fool your body. You'll end up doing what is right for you. If you want to review how intensity should be estimated, you can go to the Modified Borg-Noble Intensity Scale in Appendix C.

One of the great aspects of L.E.A.P. is that it shows you what your own individual goals should be and where your boundaries lie. There is great flexibility in being able to define levels, zones, and boundaries on an individual basis. There is always a physical activity level that is right for you, and L.E.A.P. allows you to work at that level and helps you stay within your limits. L.E.A.P. allows you to be in charge of your physical activity.

Now let's go through some common questions using a what-if format and a desire to reach the optimal ECPs level as the goal.

"WHAT IF I DON'T REACH MY OPTIMAL LEVEL?"

Nobody can always reach their optimal level. We all have other things that sometimes divert our best intentions. As I said, we all have grandmothers that come to visit. We all have somebody that needs help. We all have deadlines we can't miss. The reason I put zones of accomplishment in L.E.A.P. is to let you know that not reaching your optimal level is no reason to become discouraged and no reason to feel you have failed. The different zones and levels show you that physical activity has still been a positive force in your life during the week.

If you don't reach your optimal EPCs for the week but do reach the risk reduction level, you should feel good that you reached this first plateau of success. You are doing more physical activity than 80% of the people in America.

Reaching the risk reduction level insures that you are doing enough physical activity so that it is a positive factor in your life. This is the level of energy conversion that the American Medical Association recommends as the least you should do to gain benefits from physical activity. There is significant value in your risk reduction ECPs.

If your Week 1 Optimal ECPs are below the risk reduction level, be patient and work toward that level according to the guidelines in the Progression Program. It shouldn't take long to get there.

If you exceed the risk reduction level but do not reach your optimal zone, you are in your success zone. You are doing more physical activity than at least 80% of the people in America. If you find yourself in your success zone week after week, you should consider that you have made physical activity a part of your life. If everyone was in their physical activity success zone, most of our country's medical problems and expenses would disappear. Other levels that you can aim at, which may be below your optimal level, are the body change level and the VO2Max level. Each step along the way is a brick in your fitness wall.

Your optimal ECPs goal resides in the middle of your optimal zone. You need not hit this goal exactly on the nose. If you reach your optimal zone each week, you are one of the few people in the entire United States that are doing what is physically best for themselves.

"WHAT IF I EXCEED MY OPTIMAL ZONE?"

Sometimes you may exceed your optimal zone for the week. Should you feel you did even better than expected? Should you feel this will make you even fitter? No! You have an optimal zone of energy conversion. Exceeding that zone means you are doing too much. You cannot sustain this level of energy conversion. When you are in your overtraining zone, the probability that you will become ill, injured, or emotionally bored with physical activity significantly increases. After a period of time this level of physical activity brings you to Selye's exhaustion stage.

The zones and your position in them are an example of the flexibility of L.E.A.P. L.E.A.P. enables you to respond promptly to your activity accomplishments, problems, and questions.

OTHER WHAT-IF QUESTIONS

Here are some other questions that demonstrate L.E.A.P.'s versatility in figuring out what to do. Some of the answers are based on knowing two of the three unknowns in the ECPs formula.

Let's say Marlene knows how many ECPs she wants to earn and how much time she has to do the physical activity. She needs to find out how hard she needs to work. The question is:

- "What if I want to earn 40 ECPs by riding a bike for 35 minutes? How hard will I have to ride?"

The answer is about 80 %VO2Max. This is how she got the answer.

$$ECPs = VO_2MaxWgt_{Coef} \times Duration \times I_{Coef}$$

She knows:

Her VO2MaxWgtCoef = 1.58
She wants to earn 75 ECPs.
She has 35 minutes to ride.

She wants to find out at what intensity she should ride.

75 = 1.58 x 35 x ICoef
Icoef= 75 ÷ (1.58 x 35) = 1.36

This is an Intensity Coefficient that equates to almost 80% VO2Max. At this level of intensity Marlene would feel the challenge of the physical activity to be strong, her breathing would be deep, but steady, and it would be difficult for her to talk.

- "What if it's the last day of the week and I've already reached my optimal ECPs level?"

The best physical activity you can do is no physical activity. You are at your optimal level. That's where your body wants to be for this week.

- "What if it's the last day of the week and I have less than 40% of my ECPs left to reach my optimal level. How do I figure out how to reach my optimal ECPs level?"

If you have less than 40% of your ECPs remaining, you can reach your optimal level by selecting a duration or intensity and then figuring out the unknown. You already know how many ECPs you need.

Example

Optimal Level	= 324
40% ECPs	= 130
Current Total ECPs	= 227
ECPs Remaining	= 97

This is less than 40%, so Marlene can earn all of them. She wants to ride a bike and feels like working out at 85% VO2Max (ICoef 1.62).

Duration = 97 ECPs ÷ (1.58 x 1.62) = 38 minutes

If Marlene rides for about 38 minutes, she will come very close to reaching her optimal level for the week.

With ECPs there is no guessing. You know what is right for you.

- "What if it's the last day of the week and I have more than 40% of my ECPs left to reach my optimal level? How do I figure out how to reach my optimal level?"

This week you don't reach it. Don't go over 40% of your optimal level in any one day.

Example

Optimal Level	= 324
40% ECPs	= 130
Current Total ECPs	= 151
ECPs Remaining	= 172

172 ECPs are more than 40%; Marlene can earn no more than 130 ECPs. If she still wants to ride a bike but only wants to work at an intensity of 70% VO2Max (ICoef 1.00), how long can she ride?

Duration = 130 ECPs ÷ (1.58 x 1.00) = 82 minutes

Marlene can ride for 1 hour and 22 minutes at that intensity and stay under 40% of her optimal ECPs.

In fact, 40% of your optimal ECPs is quite a bit of energy conversion at one time. Marlene, in this example, would be foolish to try to earn all 172 ECPs remaining. She could do it, but chances are very good that she would become ill or injured in the near future. The 130 ECPs still puts Marlene well into her success zone and insures that she does not go over the 40% limit for one day. Staying within her ability to convert energy will allow her to continue her physical activity program next week and make physical activity a part of her life.

Knowing what your goals are alerts you promptly when you have done too much in a day or a week. Knowing this allows you to remedy the situation immediately. If you earn over 40% of your weekly goal in one day, you should simply take the next day off (the hard day-easy day principle) to insure that you recover from the excess conversion of energy.

- "What if I have a choice of doing something short and hard or long and easy? Which is better?"

In general, it doesn't matter. What matters is that you consistently convert the energy via physical activity. Let's say Marlene wanted to earn 63 ECPs. She could vary the duration and intensity anyway she wanted.

At 70% VO2Max Marlene would have to work out for 40 minutes.

$$63 \text{ ECPs} \div (1.58 \times 1.00) = 40 \text{ minutes}$$

At about 78% VO2Max Marlene would have to work out for 30 minutes.

$$63 \text{ ECPs} \div (1.58 \times 1.33) = 30 \text{ minutes}$$

At about 85% VO2Max Marlene would have to work out for 25 minutes.

$$63 \text{ ECPs} \div (1.58 \times 1.60) = 25 \text{ minutes}$$

To earn 63 ECPs she would have to work out longer at a lower intensity than if she worked out at a higher intensity. Though it would take more minutes to make progress at a lower intensity, it would be safer. By working at a higher intensity she would make progress in fewer total minutes, but she might need longer to recover and the risk of injury would increase.

If she wanted to improve speed or strength or her ability to tolerate lactate, she might work even shorter and harder, between 90% and 95% VO2Max. She should only work at this high intensity after she has been active for a 13-week cycle and knows her body can handle the load.

- "What if I don't have much time, but I still want to earn the ECPs I need?"

It would probably be better to choose an activity that was continuous in nature, like walking, jogging, swimming, or cycling. The continuous nature of the activity, as opposed to the stop-and-go nature of basketball where there are breaks, allows you to score more ECPs in a given time at the same intensity.

For example, if Marlene jogged for 30 minutes at 75% VO2Max she would earn 57 ECPs.

$$1.58 \times 30 \text{ min} \times 1.20 = 57 \text{ ECPs}$$

If she played basketball for 30 minutes, even though at times her %VO2Max might be near 90, when she considered the breaks in the action she might well feel her overall average %VO2Max was 65. She would earn 18 fewer ECPs from the same time spent playing basketball.

$$1.58 \times 30 \text{ min} \times .82 = 39 \text{ ECPs}$$

In this example, to earn 57 ECPs in basketball she would have to play for 44 minutes.

$$57 \text{ ECPs} \div (1.58 \times .82) = 44 \text{ min}$$

- "What if I haven't reached my optimal zone for the week? If I have chosen the Progression Program, how do I progress next week?"

If you have reached your optimal zone, your progression

is as you originally figured it out. If you haven't reached your optimal zone, you ended in one of three places:

1: You did not reach your success zone.

Rule: If you did not reach your success zone, go back to the optimal level of 3 weeks ago.

Wherever you are in your program, go back 3 weeks. This means that if in Week 5 you did not reach your success zone, your optimal level for Week 6 is the same as it was for Week 2 (Week 5 – 3 Weeks = Week 2).

2: You are in your success zone but are closer to your risk reduction level than you are to your optimal level.

Rule: If you are in your success zone but are closer to your risk reduction level than your optimal level, go back 2 weeks.

Wherever you are in your program, go back 2 weeks. This means that if in Week 5 you are in your success zone but are closer to your risk reduction level than you are to your optimal level, your optimal level for Week 6 is the same as it was for Week 3 (5 – 2).

3: You are in your success zone and are closer to your optimal level than you are to your risk reduction level.

Rule: If you are in your success zone and are closer to your optimal level than your risk reduction level, go back 1 week."

Wherever you are in your program, go back 1 week. This means that if in Week 5 you are in your success zone and are closer to your optimal level than you are to your risk reduction level, your optimal level for Week 6 is the same as it was for Week 4 (5 – 1).

Each of these choices involves redoing your 13-Week Progression chart. It is worth the effort because it allows your progression goal to correspond with your body's ability to adapt and progress.

This is how the second situation, being in her success zone but closer to her risk reduction level than to her optimal level, might cause Marlene's 13-Week Progression cycle to change:

Week 1 ECPs	= 324
ECPs Increase	= 3
Risk Reduction	= 126
ECPs for Week 5	= 150 (150 is closer to 126 than to 324)

Table 13.2

Week #	Optimal Goal Cycle #1		Actual Cycle #1
1	324		319
2	327		322
3	330		334
4	333		329
5	336		**150**
6	~~339~~	330	
7	~~342~~	333	
8	~~345~~	336	
9	~~348~~	339	
10	~~351~~	342	
11	330		
12	318		
13	0		

After Week 5, where Marlene did not reach her optimal level, Week 6 has been adjusted back to the optimal level of Week 3 (you are in your success zone but are closer to your risk reduction level than to your optimal level; go back 2 weeks). Weeks 11 and 12 always stay the same as they originaly were.

- "What if I do too much and end up in the overtraining zone?"

If you earn enough ECPs to put you in the overtraining zone, add the optimal level for the week in which you overtrained to that of the following week. Then subtract the ECPs you earned in the week you overtrained from the total of the 2 weeks. This will be your goal for the next week. Then you can pick up your progression without further adjustments.

Here's an example of how Marlene should adjust her progression if she finishes in the overtraining zone in Week 5:

Week 1 ECPs	= 324
ECPs Increase	= 3
Risk Reduction	= 126
Overtraining Zone	= 348
ECPs for Week 5	= 364 (Marlene is 40 ECPs above optimal)

Goal Week 6= (336 + 339) – 364 = 675 – 364 = 311

Marlene's goal for Week 6 is 311 ECPs.

Table 13.3

Week #	Optimal Goal Cycle #1	Actual Cycle #1
1	324	319
2	327	322
3	330	334
4	333	329
5	336	~~354~~ 364
6	~~339~~ 311	
7	342	
8	345	
9	348	
10	351	
11	354	
12	330	
13	318	

If you don't respect overtraining, you will not make physical activity a consistent, effective part of your life.

I had a friend who never worked out. He was overweight and not very vigorous. I convinced him to begin the L.E.A.P. program. After about 6 months he had lost a significant amount of fat, gained a significant amount of muscle, and was feeling very, very good about his health, himself, and his life. One weekend he went cross-country skiing and, in addition to completing his ECPs goal for the week ending on Saturday, he got so many points on Sunday that he completed his goal for the upcoming week also. When he got back he called me and told me how happy he was to have felt so good skiing and all about the ECPs he had earned. I told him he should take the rest of the week off because he had already done what was in his best interests physically. Of course he didn't, because he was feeling so good. About 2 weeks later he was puzzled that he was suddenly feeling very tired and very unmotivated. He even had a cold. It took me some time to convince him of the connection between his lethargy/cold and overdoing the physical activity. It took him a long time to get back to a physical activity program.

- "What if I was significantly under my optimal level the first 2 weeks, but I feel I'm doing as much as I can?"

Use the 2-week fine-tune reset number. Add the ECPs you earned from Week 1 and Week 2 and divide by 2. Use that as your new optimal level, and make a new 13-Week Progression schedule based on the new number.

- "What if I was significantly over my optimal level the first 2 weeks, but it was easy for me?"

Add the ECPs from Week 1 to Week 2 and divide by 2. Use that as your new optimal level, and make a new 13-Week Progression schedule based on the new number.

- "What if something changes in my life that will improve my ability to convert energy?"

You can go back to the autobiography anytime you want. If you think you can earn more ECPs, going back to the autobiography shows you how far ahead you can safely advance.

- "What if I worked out harder than I planned one day, but I have a hard workout planned the next day?"

As long as you don't earn more than 66% of your optimal level in 2 days, you will normally be all right because you will have the 5 other days to do 33% of your optimal level.

- "What if I don't feel 100%. Should I be physically active?"

You should listen to what your body is trying to tell you. Sometimes you may just feel tired, and being physically active will help rather than hurt. Other times the worst thing you can do is go for a workout. I've interpreted some easy-to-understand messages the body sends that can help you know what to do. I call these messages recovery indicators. Every morning they can tell you if your body has recovered from recent challenges. It takes about 2 minutes. After you check these indicators for 2 weeks to get averages, you can start using them.

Here's what you do:

1: Just before you get out of bed, estimate the hours of sleep you got. You may have gone to bed at 10 P.M. and are getting out of bed at 6 A.M., but you may not have slept all that time. Just make a good honest estimate of how many hours you believe you slept. If the figure you get is within 10% of the average you have probably gotten enough sleep. You've given your body enough of an opportunity to recover.
2: Then, still in bed, take a 1-minute pulse rate. If your pulse rate is no higher than 10% above normal, it's a good sign that you have recovered.
3: Finally, get out of bed, go to the bathroom, and void. Then weigh yourself naked. If you are 97% of your normal body weight or higher, you've probably rehydrated and renourished your body properly.

What do you do if you have had less than 90% of your normal sleep, your heart rate is more than 110% of normal, and your body weight is more than 3% below normal?

1: If one of these recovery indicators is off, it's probably OK to be physically active, but if you don't feel very well after you start exercising, be prepared to stop the workout or at least reduce its duration and intensity.
2: If two indicators are abnormal, do less than planned and don't work at an intensity above 60% VO2Max.
3: If all three recovery indicators are abnormal, take the day off.

- "What if I have cold or flu symptoms or am sick?"

The best advice is to not work out. Your body is fighting a battle with some invader. It is converting energy trying to overcome that challenge. If you do work out, you may feel better for a short time during and immediately after the physical activity. You won't be as hot, and you'll feel somewhat exhilarated, the way you do when you get a good workout. But what has really happened is that you've put your body in an awkward position. Part of it says it has to fight the flu; another part says it has to supply blood to contracting muscles. The blood to the contracting muscles wins because it is the most immediate problem. It's the squeaky wheel saying, "Choose me, choose me!" Meanwhile the viruses are saying, "Wow! Did this guy quit, or what? All of a sudden there are fewer white cells." So the viruses bulk up, and within a few hours after your workout is over the battle with them is raging again.

If you feel sick, it is best not to work out. Let your body address itself to fighting whatever is invading it. If the illness lasts more than 3 days, I have another rule of thumb. Don't start working out again until you have felt 100% well for 24 straight hours. When you do start again, it's best to complete the week at a reduced level of intensity. Then when a new week arrives, use the rules we spoke about earlier

- "What if I'm not ill but injured?"

What type of injury is it? If your exercise is running and you sprained your right wrist, you can run. If you're a right-handed tennis player and you sprained your right wrist, it would probably be better if you allowed it to rest. The point is that you don't want to aggravate an injury. Rule of thumb: If the injury doesn't feel as if it's gone after 3 to 5 minutes of the activity, you should stop!

- "What if I'm not ill, but I have a lot of emotional overloads. Should I still work out?"

It would probably be a great idea to get in a short work-out because working out gives the stress a place to go. You'll probably feel you're in a better position to handle the stress after you have a workout than you were before.

When I was working on my doctorate I was between forty-five and fifty-two years of age. I had to work hard to remember what my younger peers had little problem remembering. So test time demanded a lot of concentration. But I still made time for a short 1-mile jog each day during exams. I feel it made all the difference in my approach to the tests because I came back to the studying with renewed vigor. You don't have to work hard unless you want to. Remember, working below 60% $VO_{2}Max$ stimulates a relaxation response.

- "What if I hit a roadblock or detour and stop my physical activities for several days to several weeks or months?"

Sometimes we all hit a roadblock, a detour, or we get lost. We relapse. When this happens, what should we do? First, we should not think we are failures. Probably several factors over which we had little control contributed to the situation. Even if there were no other factors, a break in our physical activity is not cause for self-incrimination. Try to figure out why it occurred and see if there is a way you can prevent if from happening again. Maybe all it takes is making sure that physical activity is as important as any other appointment on your calendar.

Then, to figure out where you pick up your physical activity, look at how long a break you took. ECPs are flexible and provide several options for your return.

If your break was just one or two sessions, don't even look at it as a miss. You may get fewer ECPs for the week, but just pick up where you would be if you had not missed any days. Don't try to make up what you missed. That will just overload your system and insure that you will miss even more days in the near future.

Here's an example from Vicki Huber, the two-time Olympian you met in the last chapter. She has a chronic inflammatory condition in the attachment of her left Achilles tendon. Sometimes it flares up and she has to take a day or two off. When she comes back she has one easy day and then can usually get back on schedule. Table 13.4 shows how she modifies her workouts.

Table 13.4

Day	Planned (in minutes)	Actual (in minutes)
Sunday	110	110
Monday	50	50
Tuesday	75	**missed**
Wednesday	50	**missed**
Thursday	50	easy **30**
Friday	50	50
Saturday	75	75
	500	315

Vicki does not try to make up the days she missed. It is more important to make sure her Achilles will not immediately flare up again. She only runs a little more than 60% of her planned week, but she comes out of the week ready to train fully again the following week and not still nursing a sore Achilles.

If you have been physically inactive for 1 to 2 weeks, you can either restart your physical activity at Week 1 of the 13-week cycle or go back 3 weeks and restart from there. Don't go back to a previous 13-week cycle.

Let's use Marlene as an example. Recently she took a short vacation with her daughter. She was gone 10 days and was in Week 6 when she left. Here's how her 13-week cycle looked.

Table 13.5

Week #	Optimal Goal Cycle #1		Actual Cycle #1
1	324		319
2	327		322
3	330		334
4	333		329
5	336		336
6	339		
	vacation		
7	342		vacation
8	~~345~~	330	
9	~~348~~	333	
10	~~351~~	336	
11	330		
12	318		
13	0		

When Marlene started her program again, her optimal level was the same as in Week 3. There was no need to change Weeks 11 and 12.

If you have been gone for longer than 2 weeks, it probably would be a good idea to redo your autobiography or start at the beginning of the 13-week cycle previous to the one you were in before you had the detour. Roadblocks and detours don't mean you can't find a way to reach your goal of making physical activity a part of your life.

- "What if my job requires physical labor. Should I still work out?"

Caloric expenditure is dependent upon many personal and environmental factors. The table below shows, in general, comparisons between the physical activities involved in different occupations and forms of exercise. Cross-country skiing is arbitrarily given a 10. Remember, these are very general and are included to give you an idea of what various physical activities demand with respect to each other. If you are in an occupation whose score is equal to or greater than 4.0, you are probably getting enough physical activity in a gravity environment and might consider doing water activities to relieve pressure on bones, cartilage, and joints, while at the same time getting some aerobic work.

Table 13.6

Physical Activity	Score
Lying at ease	1.5
Office Work	2.0
Baking/Cooking	2.5
Sewing	3.0
Clerking/Counter Work	3.5
Driver	3.5
Housekeeping	3.5
Electrician	4.0
Machine Tooling	4.0
Golf	4.0
Building/Painting	5.0
Walking	5.0
Warehousing	5.5
Farming	5.5
Cycling	6.0
Tennis	6.5
Forestery	7.5
Shoveling/Mill Work	8.5
Swimming	9.0
Running	9.5
Cross-country Skiing	10.0

If you have a job that demands physical labor and want to be active in addition to your job, that's OK. But to make sure you do not overdo, you should include your work as a physical activity in the Current Physical Activity section of your autobiography. And when you are active, you should do activities that are different from what you do at work. If you deliver mail, you probably get enough aerobic exercise, but you may want to supplement that with strength, flexibility, and water activities.

If you are lugging boxes around all day in a warehouse, you might want to stay away from strength work but do some stretching and water running. Once again, the water will help modify the effects of gravity and can give you a nice aerobic workout. As always, games are fun and a great way to get away from it all.

- "What if I want to have sexual relations the night before a hard workout or athletic contest. Will it hurt my performance?"

It shouldn't, because the energy conversion is not usually excessive. It might even be beneficial because of the relaxation and positive feelings it provides. One of the athletes I coach was able to stay with her husband the night before her final event in the Olympics and they conceived their first child that night. She had the best overall result of any U.S. competitor the next day. Casey Stengel, the Hall of Fame baseball manager, summed it up well when he said, "It's not sex that's the problem, it's staying up all night looking for it."

- "What if I want a program that will produce the best overall results?"

This depends on the level you are at and where you want to go. Each individual is different. But any program like this would combine an aerobic activity, a balanced strength activity, and some stretching. You might include a game you enjoy several days a week.

• "What if I want to do the best physical activities I can?"

The best physical activities for you are the ones that are fun. The next best might be activities that serve a dual purpose, such as working around the house or riding a bike to the store to get something. The next best might be some rhythmical endurance activities like walking, jogging, or running. Strength activities done properly can give you both a strength and an aerobic benefit. Maintaining your strength is very important. And don't forget flexibility. It's a tough question to answer, because there are so many individual goals and aspects to being physically fit.

• "What if my intensity is between numbers on the Modified Borg–Noble Intensity Scale?"

When using this scale it is all right to interpolate between the listed coefficents. For example, if you believe your intensity was 73% VO2Max, you could use 1.12 as your ICoef, which is between 1.00 (70%) and 1.20 (75%) on the Modified Borg-Noble Scale.

CHAPTER 14

"WHAT IF I KEEP COMING UP WITH EXCUSES?"

With L.E.A.P. many of the excuses are invalid. If you can't make your optimal level, and sometimes we can't, L.E.A.P. has provided alternate goals that still enable you to benefit from physical activity. All L.E.A.P. wants you to do is try to put physical activity into your life. The risk reduction level is much better than inactivity.

- "I don't know what to do."

L.E.A.P. provides tools you can always fall back upon when you have questions about where to begin; how often, how long, and how hard to work; how to progress and how to measure progression; how to react to changes in your life or in you; how to plan a schedule and change it based on what happened yesterday or today or what will happen tomorrow; and what to do when you miss some days on which you planned to be physically active.

L.E.A.P. acts as a mentor by providing simple guidelines upon which you will be able to make flexible, accurate, informed, and individual decisions. Anyone with an experienced mentor by their side has a much better chance of understanding what they are doing.

A mentor helps you know yourself and understand how your personal demographics, health habits, lifestyle, and current physical activity pattern affect your position on the health continuum. From this biographical information a mentor helps you determine your location on a fitness map and establish a destination, or goal. The goal is up to you but to a certain extent is restricted. Choosing a goal that is unrealistic is inviting failure. A mentor prevents this by helping you pick goals you can actually achieve and recognizes that goals can be flexible, especially at the beginning. Goals should be reevaluated as you learn more about yourself and physical activity.

Once a goal has been established, a good mentor will help you by suggesting routes you might consider taking to your goal. The mentor also understands that as you meet the challenges of your physical goal, you need to balance the challenges with recovery. A mentor will help you evaluate what you have done and put into perspective how that affects progress toward your goal. If the mentor sees that changes to your route may be appropriate, those changes will be suggested.

Having a mentor insures that you have objective guidance nearby, guidance that will help you make crucial and realistic decisions for yourself. L.E.A.P. acts as a mentor. You will know what to do.

• "It's not convenient."

The complaint "It's not convenient" with respect to location deserves to be respected. Getting there may take some effort, and getting there may seem like an intrusion. Being there may cost something.

What may help overcome the inconvenience is to examine the opportunities for an "anchor location." In real estate they say the three most important qualities of a property are location, location, and location. An anchor location should be a physical and emotional location that you look forward to going to and being in. The environment should be pleasing to you, and the people should be friendly, supportive, and sensitive to your needs and personality. It doesn't have to be the fanciest place in town. You don't have to have a socially accepted location. It's more important that it be a location you can access on a regular basis. There are health clubs in every city and town that are within convenient distance of where you live or work. The financial investment required to join most clubs is worth the return. You will find it easier if the place is clean and has a place to change and shower. It's helpful to have some equipment or court space that is accessible at the time you want to use it and that you enjoy using. And it would be good to have access to out-of-doors walking, jogging, or biking opportunities.

An anchor location need not be a club. It can be where you live. Instead of investing in a membership, maybe you can use that money to develop some space where you can be active at home or from which you have access to some good running or biking trails. The place you work, especially if a shower is available, can serve as your anchor location.

An anchor location need not be a permanent place. It can be a league in which you participate in some type of game. An anchor location can be a place you pass by on your way to or from your job. A friend of mine runs 3 miles a day in Eugene on the Amazon Trail, a running trail in the center of town. He changes at work, gets in his car, and starts to drive home. His way home takes him past the trail. When he gets there he parks and runs his 3 miles. Then he gets in his car and goes home. Sometimes he runs hard, but his attitude about the running is relaxed. For example, if the temperature is above 75, he only runs 2 miles. If it is above 90, he runs 1 mile. He carries a towel and jacket in his car in case it is raining. When he finishes he goes home and takes a shower. Maybe the whole thing takes 25 to 30 minutes, but what a great investment of time. He has something to look forward to every day. He knows he will get his physical activity in every day. He knows how good he feels after he accomplishes his goal of being physically active. In the '50s and '60s great Olympic runners had full-time jobs. The location of their physical activity was very often the route they took running to and from work.

A reminder. Perhaps the single most important thing about an anchor location, if it is not where you live or work, is that it should be a sanctuary or a place you look forward to going. Being there should give you a good feeling. Maybe it is the location or the environment or the people. You should like being in your anchor location.

What I hope you see is that "convenience" is only limited by your imagination. If you want to make activity a part of your life, you will find a place to be active.

• "Nobody cares if I'm physically active or not."

The first thing I think when I hear this is "What's important is that you care."

The second thing I think about is the movie *Field of Dreams* and the line "If you build it, they will come." If your physical activity does not significantly interfere with your other responsibilities and if you seem more healthy and alive, family, friends, and employers who may not have been supportive at the beginning will often begin to encourage your efforts and end up becoming very supportive. They may even join you in some of your physical activities. At the very least, they will respect your efforts. They might even be envious.

You can take an active role in helping this happen. Sharing with them why you want to make physical activity a part of your life is a good place to start. When you try to change, people around you wonder why. They may wonder how this will affect them and become uneasy about the situation. If you communicate your reasons and thoughts, you may be able to win over someone who is doubtful or who opposes your desire to be more physically active. Bringing them into your confidence can only help if they are people who care about you.

When you start to reap the beneficial effects of a physical activity habit that is right for you, you will earn their respect, if not their full support. Respect never hurts. They may even start to wonder if they might successfully add physical activity to their lives. If you are not evangelistic, you might be able to help them by sharing some of your experiences. Sharing some of these insights can also help you solidify your physical activity habit.

Another benefit of letting family, friends, or employers know what you are trying to do is that they unwittingly become an active support network. Even if they never talk to you about what you are doing, you have made a commitment to yourself that they know about. It's harder to break a commitment when others know what you have committed to. Also, knowing what you are trying to accomplish, they may be more inclined to make supportive comments or gestures that encourage you in the difficult times when you may think physical activity isn't for you that particular day. It may be just that one comment from a family member, friend, or employer that gets you through the next workout. That workout could be the one that gets you to your habit.

You can also actively seek support groups. Being on a team is a guaranteed way to find several people that like the same thing you do and will be supportive of your efforts. Many health clubs now keep lists of people that share similar interests. Entering a race or tournament is another way to build a support network. Support is available. You may have to build it or find it. But it's there.

• "I don't have control over my life."

This excuse always reminds me of the person who said, "I'd like to talk to the person in charge of my life and suggest some changes." Sometimes it seems hard to understand that the responsibility is ours.

Business, in its desire to sell, and government, in its desire to help or control, too often send a message that seems to say, "Let us help!" but subliminally says, "Don't worry. Put your faith in us and give us your money. We'll take it from there!" TV news says, "We'll inform you." Hollywood says, "We'll entertain you." Fast food franchises say, "We'll feed you." Shoe companies say, "We'll dress you."

It's easy in this busy world to succumb to the subtle messages from the public relations and advertising industry that tell us they have the answers and they can solve our problems. "A Little Dab'll Do Ya." In a speech he made several years ago, comedian Dick Gregory was talking about the caffeine, tobacco, alcohol, drugs, fast food, and junk food that we put into our bodies. He was describing how we are blinded to the real impact of these products by advertising, which usurps responsibility by telling us what we like to hear rather than what we need to hear. He said:

> But if I was telling you about some gas that would mess up your car, immediately you wouldn't put it in no more. They have reduced us down to such an insignificant nothing that we have more respect for our automobiles, we have more respect for our wardrobes, than we have for ourselves.

From the health care/fitness industry, insurance companies, HMOs, health clubs, health product manufacturers, and many physicians, the message is very similar: "Let us take care of your problems. We have the answer. Don't ask too many questions, just let us handle it."

L.E.A.P. provides you with the powerful tools you need in order to accept responsibility for your physical activity. L.E.A.P. empowers you with the ability to determine a place to start, a physical activity goal, and routes to follow. And L.E.A.P. gives you a clear way to measure your progress so that you can say to yourself, "I'm taking care of myself. I'm handling myself. And it has consequences that I can see and feel. I feel good about myself."

- "It's OK after I'm out there, but it's hard to begin the activity."

If you feel like this, you're not unusual. The first step or motion of the physical activity may be the hardest one you'll take. Often the first step is the one you take even before you have your workout gear on. It's the one where you make the commitment to work out, the one where you pick up your workout gear and go out the door. Remember Australian Ron Clarke, a multiple world record holder in distance running, who said the hardest part of his workout was "to put on me shorts and get out the door."

It's like inertia—it takes more energy to get a mass moving that it does to keep it moving. Sometimes you're working on a project or watching TV, it's raining out, or your club is a few miles away. It's so much easier to stay put. Taking the first step takes a lot of mental energy. But once you make the first step, the physical activity is almost a sure thing. Once you're active, completing your workout is easy.

Almost every athlete I've ever coached faces the same challenge. It's hard to get started. That's why it is so important to make a commitment that you will not rationalize away the first step. If you still don't want to work out after you have your shorts on and are out the door, then turn around and come home. That's OK. I'll bet you will rarely turn around.

- "I don't have enough time!"

The time you invest in physical activity doesn't have to be excessive, but it must become a consistent part of your life. Remember the CEO that said that making time for physical activity was as important to him as any other appointment on his calendar. I want you to take it a step further. It is *more* important than any appointment on your calendar. To enhance the opportunity for a long life filled with quality years, physical activity is as important as eating and sleeping. You should feel, "I need to eat, I need to sleep, I need to be physically active." Thinking this way raises it another notch on the priority chart. This is where it belongs.

This is where your body places it.

Some people say, "I'll never get back the time I spend in physical activity." Actually, that's not true either. A long-term Finnish study comparing the longevity of physically active and sedentary people showed that the active people lived an average of 6 years longer than their sedentary counterparts.

The best-known study showing the relationship between physical activity and longevity was headed by Dr. Ralph Paffenbarger of Stanford University. He followed the health and mortality of 20,000 people for over 20 years. The results of the study showed that a physically active lifestyle lengthened life. His data implied that as activity increased, as measured by caloric conversion of from 500 to 3000 calories per week on physical activity, the probability of an additional 1 to 3 years of life span increased significantly.

Dr. Paffenbarger said:

> There is a longstanding belief that adequate physical activity is necessary to preserve life and its desirable qualities into old age. Discussions of this thesis date back to antiquity and have intensified in recent times. The present study adds new evidence to support this view.

You might be thinking, "What's 1 to 3 years?" What if you had 1 to 3 years right now to read or spend time with your family or to do what you wanted to do, and you had the good health to be able to do it? These years may come at the end of a lifetime, but they can still be very valuable and very enjoyable. What is more important is that all the years leading up to those additional years will be of much higher quality.

You may also be thinking, "It sounds good, but I might spend all the time represented by the additional years on physical activity, so it's a trade-off. All my additional time is really spent exercising." Even if that were true it would be time well spent. But it isn't true. As with a financial investment, you get a return on physical activity. For every hour you spend being physically active you get approximately 1.9 hours of quality life back.

Finally, the time you spend on physical activity often pays short-term benefits as well because this time may be the best personal time you get each week. In reality, you don't have enough time not to have time.

- "I'm too tired."

How do you tell if you are really too tired or are in the clutches of inertia and looking for an excuse? You get on your shorts and get out the door. If you are really too tired, your body will let you know and you can turn around and come back.

There may be times when you really are too tired. During those times it is better to pay your respects to recovery and ignore challenge. How do you know when you are really too tired? One way to tell is to use your recovery indicators, which show whether you have fully recovered from your last challenge or challenges. If your morning heart rate is 10% higher than normal, or your morning body weight is 3% less than normal, or if you slept 10% less than normal, it shows that there has been some problem with your ability to recover from the latest series of challenges, and it might be better to rest. Of course, a fever or a sore throat is always an indication that you should skip physical activity until those symptoms disappear.

But often the feeling that you're too tired can be related to the type of day you had. You may mean *tense* instead of *tired*. You may have had some deadline at work. Maybe you had a number of family responsibilities. The good news is that often when you feel tired and go ahead and engage in some physical activity, you will feel invigorated and less tired than when you started. You will also feel more relaxed. Electromyographic studies (studies of electrical activity in muscles) have repeatedly shown that physical activity reduces the tension in the muscles. Simply reducing the tension in your muscles will often be enough to make you feel less tired. Many times a workout in the middle of the day, if it can be accomplished, can increase your energy and productivity in the late afternoon. Also, an easy workout after work can help you sleep much better that evening.

Don't let a feeling of being tired deter you. You don't have to do a hard workout. But if you planned one, try to get it in. Start easy, and you may surprise yourself with how well you feel after you get a few minutes into the workout.

Dr. Herbert Benson, a medical doctor with degrees in both Western and Eastern medicine and the author of *The Relaxation Response,* has shown that easy aerobic exercise can elicit the same "relaxation response" that is elicited by meditation.

As a final thought, you should know that an investment in energy conversion, like a wise investment of dollars, can increase your resources. It does this by producing adaptation. So even when you are feeling tired, it is worth beginning the physical activity you had planned. Most times you will be pleasantly surprised with the results.

CHAPTER 15

"WHAT IF I FEEL LIKE A FAILURE BECAUSE I HAVEN'T MADE ACTIVITY A PART OF MY LIFE?"

Despite knowing how important physical activity is to your body, seeing all the benefits of L.E.A.P., and realizing how easy it is to use L.E.A.P. in your own life, you may still be having some problems motivating yourself to try it or to make it a consistent part of your life. Don't be discouraged. What you, like all of us, are trying to do with physical activity in this industrial society is to make it a habit. The bad news is that good habits are hard to form. The good news is that any habit is hard to break.

You know, whether you admit it or not, that you feel better and like yourself better when you are fit. You may already have experienced from time to time the warm glow that accompanies the completion of a reasonable physical effort. You probably feel that making physical activity a part of your life is important. It is probably one of the reasons you picked up this book in the first place.

However, chances are also good that you are one of the 45 million people in this country who want to be physically active but have not yet made physical activity a part of their life. This shouldn't depress you, because what you are trying to do—modify behavior—is very difficult. It requires repeated action until that action becomes a characteristic condition of the mind and body. Only then can it be easily and often done.

What you should realize is that wanting to do something

is already half the battle. Dr. James Prochaska has developed a six-stage model that shows people are always at different stages of readiness to change behavior:

1. Precontemplation
2. Contemplation
3. Preparation   6. Relapse
4. Action
5. Maintenance

Relapse is off to the side because it can occur anytime.

Dr. Prochaska called stage 1 *precontemplation*. In this stage you have no intention of changing behavior. In stage 2, *contemplation*, it dawns on you that a behavioral change might be good, and you begin to think about changing.

In stage 3, *preparation*, you make plans to change. Perhaps recognizing the benefit of some guidance, you see an expert or pick up a book. You may think about how to reschedule parts of your day to include regular activity. You figure out where it makes the most sense to work out. Maybe you know some people with whom you can share the physical activity. You decide what activities you would enjoy. You then try to determine how often, how long, and how hard you might work out.

You should feel good about having gotten this far but, don't stop.

Action only enters the picture at stage 4. At this stage you've committed yourself. You are putting into practice your decisions from stage 3. The stage is not that hard because you are on a "honeymoon." You are excited to be putting a plan into action.

Stage 5—*maintenance!* Here's the phase upon which your destiny rides. Anyone who seeks to make or break a habit must come face to face with maintenance. Maintenance is the time during habit formation when you must repeat the action so often that it becomes second nature and you can't imagine it not being in your life. Maintenance comes from the Latin words *manus* (hand) and *tenere* (to hold). You literally hold in your hand the success or failure of your attempt to change.

Make no mistake, you will often find yourself trying to hold onto the commitment, to continue your action in the face of an attack. The attacks often seem reasonable: family responsibilities, work commitments, feeling tired. But without being too hard on you, it needs to be said that with proper planning and an insistence in your own mind that activity is a part of life, you can fulfill work obligations, experience the joy of family interaction, and still be physically active. You may have to be less active than you want, but as you know, with L.E.A.P. there are several levels of physical activity at which you can enjoy the benefits of a physically active life.

Even more insidious attacks come from within, from your old patterns and your other self, the self of precontemplation. Look at this short scenario.

Precontemplation: You're watching a performance on TV that involves athletic stamina and dexterity. You're eating another bowl of potato chips and feeling sluggish.

Contemplation: You admire what you see, and suddenly somebody wakes up inside of you and says, "Look at yourself. You're out of shape. You're getting a little thick. Do something about it!" It's happened to all of us. Something clicks inside, and we have a different picture of who we should be.

Preparation: Soon we're cleaning out the refrigerator and restocking it with better food, or in some cases, with food. We're buying sweats and maybe some equipment, or joining a health club.

Action: Before we know it we're on a Stairmaster, in an aerobics class, or out for a long steady jog. By Monday we've lost 2 pounds. We go to sleep dreaming of running the Boston Marathon. Maybe even doing pretty well. Tuesday, another pound gone! We're incredible! Gorgeous! A lean machine! The first 2 weeks go just like this. "This isn't as hard as I thought." We keep pouring it on.

Maintenance: Then one morning when we step on the scale. . . nothing. We feel a slight twinge of resentment. But we vow to work harder. Several more experiences like this, plus maybe feeling a little more tired than we thought we would. . . and maybe missing something we long for . . . and . . .

Off the Wagon—Relapse: Somehow something has changed. The next morning the room is cold. It's also raining outside. The other person is back! And he doesn't want to run today. He doesn't even want to get out of bed. The sweats are gone. The marathon is gone. The lean machine is gone. The other guy is running the show again.

Should we give up? No. Off the wagon is just another stage, as you can see, called *relapse*. The interesting thing is that according to research, before an action can become a habit, most people go through relapse at least seven times. So again, take heart! Relapse is to be expected. What should you do when relapse strikes? Accept personal responsibility and go back to preparation. Figure out what triggered relapse and see if you can modify the effect of the trigger. Then go through the stages again. If you are perceptive and persistent, you can understand what happened, make the changes necessary, and make the individual action of engaging in physical activity into a habit that is very hard to break.

I have observed that a common cause of relapse at the beginning of a program is that people tend to overestimate the energy they are capable of spending on physical activity. They are so excited about changing their lives that they do too much, too soon, and too often. They use their available energy for too much physical activity, and the rest of their life suffers. The secret is balance. The goals, desires, and needs of the whole person must be met. For any action to become a habit, it must be structured within the framework of satisfying the reasonable goals of the whole person.

Second, and here too balance plays a role, most people don't understand how to balance challenge and recovery to attain adaptation. We are told constantly, "Go for it! Just do it!" But how to do it right is often not as clear. So we push. It's part of our culture. And very often we get ill, injured, sore, or just plain tired. And our bodies logically say, "Don't do that any more." It's not that we don't want to do the physical activity. It's that the wisdom of our own body is sending a message to tell us to slow down.

But L.E.A.P. allows you overcome these two obstacles. With L.E.A.P. you know what is exactly right and what is too much. You also know that built into L.E.A.P. is the automatic balance of challenge and recovery.

When the change you sought is now a habit, your desire to retain physical activity in your life will usually be stronger than the desire to return to a more sedentary lifestyle. With L.E.A.P. making sure you're doing what is right for you, you will be able to make physical activity a lifelong passion.

CHAPTER 16

"WHAT IF I WANT TO LOSE WEIGHT?"

You approach the problem of weight loss by first forgetting about weight loss. Second, you learn about the muscle-to-fat ratio. Losing weight is not just a matter of losing pounds. Real weight control is working toward the highest ratio of healthy muscle tissue to fat tissue you can attain. Everyone has a ratio that is right for them.

I coach a lot of wonderful female athletes. Sometimes when we start working together they ask, "Coach, what should I weigh?" I say, "I don't know. If you train consistently and eat an intelligent diet, you will weigh what you are supposed to weigh at the right time. Don't worry about weight. Focus on training and eating properly." The same is true for everyone. If you make physical activity a part of your life and eat intelligently, your body will automatically balance itself at the right ratio.

FORGET WEIGHT LOSS! Weight loss is a cash cow. The diet industry spends billions on advertising that aims at your weight loss vanity button. The publishing industry takes in billions to publish the advertising for weight loss systems and products. We as consumers spend billions on weight loss vanity-enhancing products. Most of the products are superficial, overpriced, and ineffective. *Forget weight loss!* Concentrating on weight loss alone usually changes a person from someone who is physically weak and overweight to someone who is physically weak and not as overweight and who will gain the weight back. *Consumer Reports,* in a survey of almost every contemporary diet-only program, found that all the weight that was lost was gained back within 2 years.

REMEMBER MUSCLE-TO-FAT RATIO! Concentrating on the muscle-to-fat ratio usually changes a person from someone who is physically weak and overweight to someone who is stronger and healthier and looks better. A physically active lifestyle based on L.E.A.P. will be the most effective regimen you can use to help you reach and maintain your best muscle-to-fat ratio for a lifetime.

The reason a higher muscle-to-fat ratio is important is found in the characteristics of the two tissues. Muscle is more active than fat, so it converts energy at a much higher rate, nine times as fast per pound. Muscle is more dense than fat, so it doesn't take up as much space. It is more attractive than fat because it has shape and tone.

Fat (from an Old English word meaning "to cram") is a connective tissue found under the skin and around organs. It is made up of fat cells. It is an evolutionary storehouse for energy that was needed when we were tied more closely to seasons. Even though it is still a very important tissue, too much of it is detrimental. Having too much fat is probably the leading cause of death among adults in the industrial world. For one thing, your heart must work harder to pump blood through the extra mile of capillaries in every pound of fat.

There are two types of fat, white and brown. White fat is an effective insulator. Brown fat, also found in humans, is not a good insulator, but it is a good heat generator. Bears have brown fat, which they convert in the winter when they hibernate. Thinner people have a higher percentage of brown fat than overweight people. Overweight people have extensive reserves of white fat. One result of ignoring the Law of Conservation of Energy is that energy is converted to white fat.

If you are sedentary and eat a poor diet, your muscle-to-fat ratio will be lower and your health and appearance will be poorer than if you are physically active and eat a good diet.

You can easily figure out what's happening to your muscle-to-fat ratio by weighing yourself once, pinching yourself twice, then dividing your weight by the sum of the two pinches. It's easy. It's also less expensive than and about as informative as other methods of determining how muscle tissue compares to fat tissue in your body. You don't have to compare yourself with other people. It gives you great information. It gives you the relative change in your muscle-to-fat ratio from successive measurements. At home, in privacy, you can see how this ratio is changing anytime you want.

I have seen many people measured for body composition by many different methods. I have performed underwater weighings on over 300 people to determine their percentage of fat. I have used calipers to measure seven sites on athletes for over 20 years. I believe that using the method I describe will give you just as valuable and perhaps more practical information than any other body composition measurement.

You can buy calipers if you want, but you could also use a ruler. All you have to do is this.

1: Weigh yourself.
Hint: Make sure you weigh yourself at the same time of day when you are doing a muscle-to-fat ratio. The best time to weigh yourself is in the morning as soon as you get out of bed, after you void, before you have eaten, and with no clothes on.
2: On your abdomen, next to your belly button, pinch the skin with your thumb and index finger. Pinch so the fold of skin you raise is perpendicular to the floor. With a ruler, measure or have someone measure for you the distance between your thumb and index finger.
3: On your side, above the top of your hip bone, pinch the skin between your thumb and index finger. This time the fold of skin you pinch should be angled 45 degrees to the floor. Measure the thickness of the skinfold.

Hint: You can use either metric or English units. It doesn't matter as long as you do it the same way each time you measure. Try to take the pinches at the same time of day and pinch the same place each time. Different people put on fat at different places. But as we mature, fat seems to collect around the abdomen and hips in most of us. So these are two convenient, valid sites to pinch. You can choose other sites if you wish or do more than two. These are your numbers and only meaningful to you.

4: Add the two pinch numbers together and divide that number into your body weight.

Bingo! You have a muscle-to-fat ratio. Don't compare it with anyone else's ratio. Each time you get the ratio, compare it with your last measurement. If the ratio is higher, your fat-free weight has increased. If it is lower, your fat weight has increased. It's simple, direct, and honest.

What's important is how you are changing relative to yourself, not how you compare with others. Each person is different, and each of us has a muscle-to-fat ratio at which we function best. Our bodies will let us know where that is.

If your muscle-to-fat ratio has increased, no matter what has happened to your weight, the *percentage* of muscle tissue in your body has increased. This is good! More muscle converts more energy, improves your health, and makes you look better.

Example

Marlene's 1st Measurement

Weight	= 143 pounds
Pinches	= 1.5 inches
Muscle-to-Fat Ratio	= 95.3

Marlene's 2d Measurement

Weight	= 145 pounds
Pinches	= 1.25 inches
Muscle-to-Fat Ratio	= 116.0

Marlene gained 2 pounds but lost .25 inches in pinches, and her muscle-to-fat ratio increased from 95.3 to 116.0. That meant that the percentage of muscle tissue in her body had increased.

If the ratio has decreased, no matter what has happened to the weight, the percentage of muscle tissue has decreased. This is not good!

Example

Marlene's 3rd Measurement

Weight	= 140 pounds
Pinches	= 1.6 inches
Muscle-to-Fat Ratio	= 87.5

This time Marlene lost weight, but her muscle-to-fat ratio decreased. Even though she lost 5 pounds, she did not improve the muscle-to-fat ratio and lost relatively more muscle tissue than fat.

In the second example Marlene gained weight, but her muscle-to-fat ratio increased. In the third, she lost weight, but her muscle-to-fat ratio decreased. Table 16.1 shows combinations of weight changes and skinfold changes resulting in muscle-to-fat ratio changes. It also shows what the results mean with respect to the ability to convert energy. The first row represents where Marlene started, and then each combination of weight and skinfold is compared with the one before it.

Table 16.1

Measurement	Body Weight	Skinfold	Muscle-to-Fat Ratio	Relative Gain In	Ability to Convert Energy
1	143	1.50	95.3		
2	145	1.25	116.0	Muscle	Improved
3	140	1.60	87.5	Fat	Reduced
4	140	1.40	100.0	Muscle	Improved
5	142	1.50	94.7	Fat	Reduced
6	143	1.25	114.4	Muscle	Improved
7	146	1.15	127.0	Muscle	Improved

Changes in Muscle-to-Fat Ratio

From this table you can see that the ability to convert energy and thereby improve health, performance, and appearance depends upon more than just weight. It depends on the type of body weight. On Marlene's last reading, her weight was actually the highest, but her skinfold was lowest, resulting in relatively more muscle tissue and an enhanced ability to convert energy.

Improving the muscle-to-fat ratio involves three energy-related factors:

1. The amount of energy ingested
2. The composition of the energy ingested
3. The amount of energy converted by physical activity

Most people associate changing weight with the concept of diet, which they understand to mean a decrease in the energy ingested. Thus they eat less, hoping to lose weight. The concept of food is a good place to start, but a real diet involves eating enough nutrient-rich food to improve the muscle-to-fat ratio. It's a very different concept from just losing weight.

Diets that emphasize weight loss alone are inefficient in improving the muscle-to-fat ratio. While it is true that these diets are low in energy, they also often lack many of the nutrients your body needs. In addition, even if these diets reduce fat tissue, they often reduce muscle tissue as well. Losing muscle tissue causes both your exercise and basal metabolic rate to slow down. This makes it harder to lose weight and even harder to keep off the weight you lose because 24 hours a day you will be converting energy at a lower rate.

Basal metabolism is the energy conversion level that sustains life. Gender, age, and height are factors affecting basal metabolism that we can't control, but we can see how these factors affect basal metabolism by comparing the basal metabolisms of a man and a woman who both weigh 150 pounds and are 5'8" tall.

As we age, our basal metabolism tends to slow down. Therefore we must be more active and eat less. What usually happens is that we are less active and eat more.

Age	Basal Metabolism	
	Male[1]	Female
25	1.18	1.08
30	1.13	1.05
40	1.10	1.03
50	1.08	1.00
60	1.04	0.97
70	0.99	0.94

Height also affects basal metabolism.

Height	Basal Metabolism	
	Male	Female
5'5"	1.15	1.05
5'8"	1.18	1.08
5'11"	1.22	1.12

---

[1] Units are calories/minute

But we can control fat-free body weight and basal metabolism through good eating habits and physical activity. As fat-free body weight increases, basal metabolism increases. Remember, fat-free body weight improvement is indicated by an increase in the muscle-to-fat ratio.

Fat-Free Weight	Basal Metabolism	
	Male	Female
110	0.94	0.90
130	1.06	0.96
150	1.18	1.08
170	1.30	1.20

Physical activity increases metabolism.

Activity	Basal Metabolism	
	Male	Female
Reclining	1.18	1.08
Sitting	1.50	1.37
Office Work	2.01	1.83
Housework	3.43	3.12
Walking	3.96	3.61
Manual Labor	5.85	5.33
Moderate Activity	6.66	6.06

Physical activity has three effects on metabolism. First, when activity levels are higher, metabolism is higher. Increasing activity converts more energy.

Second, there is a residual effect of activity. This means that after activity is completed, metabolism continues at a higher level than basal metabolism for a period of time. After a moderate jog or walk, the residual effect of the activity keeps the metabolism elevated for 50 to 75 minutes.

Third, activity increases basal metabolism, converting more energy just in the act of living because of a higher muscle-to-fat ratio. The maintenance of muscle demands more energy conversion than the maintenance of fat.

Being physically active allows you to exert considerable

control over the type and amount of weight you have. Being active is almost like a no-diet diet. In a Finnish study, overweight people were divided into two groups. One group was free to eat what they wanted and was sedentary. The other group was free to eat what they wanted but was asked to be active. The first group went from being overweight to being more overweight. The second group went from being overweight to being healthier and slimmer but still robust eaters. You can actually eat more without gaining weight. The paradox is that when you are physically active you can eat a satisfying, nutrient-rich diet and have a better muscle-to-fat ratio.

Being active may actually decrease appetite or at least make it more reliable. If you make physical activity a part of your life, when you feel hungry, you probably really are. When you are sedentary, feelings of hunger are often associated with psychological factors. When you are active it is easier to resist snacking, and when you do snack, those calories will have less of an effect.

What is the best combination of physical activity and food? With respect to physical activity the answer is simple. Reach your optimal level each week. That amount of physical activity is what is exactly right for you. More than that you won't be easily able to sustain.

For food the answer is not much more complex. Follow something like the Big Day Diet in Appendix F. If you still feel the amount of food you ingest is too much, reduce each of the handfuls of servings by about half a handful. And be patient. Think in terms of a year from now, not next week. I'll end with an example of what making just a little lifestyle change can mean in a year.

Let's say Marlene liked fast food hamburgers and fries and that she was sedentary. Let's say she wanted to increase her muscle-to-fat ratio and made a deal with herself that she'd cut out one hamburger and fries each week, plus she'd be active at her risk reduction level. Here are the numbers (we'll decrease her VO2MaxWgtCoef to .96 because in this example she is sedentary with a VO2Max of 32 ml/kg/min):

Hamburger + Fries	= 483 cal/week
483 cal x 52 weeks	= 25,116 cal/year
25,116 cal ÷ 3500 cal/lb	= 7.2 pounds not gained due to reduced intake
VO2MaxWgtCoef	= .96
ECPs/Week = .96 x 7 x 30 x .37	= 75 ECPs at risk reduction level
75 L x 4.85 cal/L	= 364 cal/week
364 cal x 48 weeks	= 17,472 calories converted per year
17,472 cal/3500 cal/lb	= 5.0 pounds not gained due to increased energy conversion

The result is that at the end of the year, all other things being equal, Marlene would weigh 12.2 pounds less than she would have had she not done the physical activity and forgone the hamburger and fries. Her muscle-to-fat ratio is also much better and contributes to her ability to convert energy all day long, making her healthier and able to perform better.

To be physically active or to eat smart? That is the question.

To be physically active and to eat smart! That is the answer!

Physical Activity + Intelligent Eating
= Improved Muscle-to-Fat Ratio
= Higher Basal Metabolism
= Health + Fitness + Appearance

The concept of changing the ratio of muscle to fat is not difficult to understand. Being physically active at the level required and eating intelligently is within reason and can be accomplished. The crucial part of the puzzle is, How much do you really want it? Where does it fit on your priority list? The choice is yours!

CHAPTER 17

FINAL NOTE: TO BE LIKE MR. RANKIN AND MR. MILLETT

Muscular vigor will always be needed to furnish the background of sanity, serenity and cheerfulness to life, to give moral elasticity to our disposition, to round off the wiry edge of fretfulness and make us good humoured and easy of approach.

William James (1892)

I met a man the other day who became a hero for me: Bob Rankin. He had flown to Eugene from San Diego to visit his granddaughter, who is an athlete I coach. He is not someone who did a heroic deed, although he may have done one at some time in his life. He is not someone who is famous or wealthy or powerful, at least to my knowledge. He is ninety-one years old, but that's nothing to be proud of in itself. Quantity without quality seems to mean little. No, it was the quality of his years that radiated through to me. He plays 18 holes of golf four times a week. His part-time housekeeper became upset with him because he was on the roof fixing a skylight. He bought a house he plans to remodel. He was a smoker until age fifty, when he read a *Reader's Digest* article that convinced him smoking was not good. That night he and his wife smoked a last cigarette and quit. He told me he couldn't die until the year 2000 because that's when his driver's license expires. And that dying on the 14th hole would be OK.

When asked, he said that his "muscular vigor" had been constant throughout his life. It didn't usually involve formal exercises as much as it did physical work around the home and participation in games he enjoyed. It seemed to furnish him with a "background of sanity, serenity, and cheerfulness to life." He was good humored and very easy to approach, and there was no trace of the "wiry edge of fretfulness" about him.

I suspect that people like Bob Rankin are heros for many of us. Maybe it's because we all aspire to live a lengthy, productive, energetic, and cheerful life. Maybe it's because we know how much better it would be if everyone possessed such a positive demeanor. Maybe it's because, in the end, we all want to die young as late as possible.

I have spoken very little about the myriad of benefits to which physical activity contributes, which give us the best chance we have to die young as late as possible. Nor need I now. One just has to look at Mr. Rankin to know what could be.

Hippocrates understood the benefits physical activity can bestow:

> All parts of the body that have a function, if used in moderation and exercised in labors in which each is accustomed, become thereby healthy, well developed, and age more slowly; but if unused and left to idle they become liable to disease, defective in growth, and age quickly.

Thomas Jefferson understood, when he wrote a letter to a young friend, Thomas Mann Randolph, in July 1787:

> With your talents and industry, with science, and that steadfast honesty which eternally pursues right, regardless of consequences, you may promise yourself

everything—but health, without which there is no happiness. An attention to health then should take place over every other object. The time necessary to secure this by active exercises, should be devoted to it in preference to every other pursuit.

Even those who don't outwardly agree that physical activity is beneficial to our health and well-being know intuitively that what Hippocrates and Jefferson said is true. Our bodies tell us. Our bodies constantly tell us in subtle and not so subtle ways that it is important for physical activity to play a balanced role in our lives.

Dr. George Sheehan made many comments about the role physical activity played in the lives of his friends, his patients, and himself. Here he describes what his body told him:

I am increasingly aware that I know more than I can tell. Much of that knowledge comes from my body. It is the body more than anything else that contributes to my feelings of certainty, or self-control, or self-esteem. . . . Your body reveals you within and without. It tells the perceptive observer your philosophy, your view of the universe.

Sometimes it seems hard for us to elevate this concept of physical activity to the place of honor it belongs. We always seem to have so much more to do. We often don't know what to do even if we make the time and overcome the inertia of getting on our shorts and getting out the door.

I know I can't force you out the door. But I wrote this book, and developed the L.E.A.P. program, because I thought it might be easier for you to get out the door if you knew what to do once you were out. I am pleased with the way L.E.A.P. turned out because it combined good science with years of practical experience to provide you with information that empowers you to develop your own lifetime exercise/activity program. It is a program that is very personal. No two L.E.A.P. programs are the same, because no two people are the same.

When I started this project 10 years ago I wanted to develop a program that you could use no matter what your age, gender, goals, or health status might be. I wanted you to be able to begin safely without tests and know what the right amount of physical activity was for you. I wanted you to be able to monitor your physical activities and respond to the feedback by making intelligent decisions that allowed you to balance the challenge of physical activity with recovery and so achieve adaptation. I wanted you to do this with your brain, your body, your desire to make physical activity a part of your life, and with this small book as an unobtrusive mentor.

Some may say this can't be done so simply. Or as some scientists might say, it can't be done "on the back of an envelope." I disagree. I started this on the back of the proverbial envelope, and while it is backed by good science to make it accurate, it is still simple to use. When people, experts included, have spent time with me one-on-one, they have all gone away agreeing that the tenets upon which the L.E.A.P. program is based are solid and provide guidance that is simple, effective, and can be trusted.

Now you have a tool that will not only enable you to "do it" but, more importantly, do it right and do it consistently! There is a huge difference between doing something and doing it correctly. Doing it right, as opposed to just doing it, is the difference between succeeding and failing. Anyone can just do it, and while the results in the beginning may be gratifying, they are usually chaotic in nature, and the period of consistent physical activity is of short duration. Doing it right increases the chances of making physical activity a part of your life.

L.E.A.P. makes it easy for you to do what organizations

concerned with health have been promoting for years: be physically active. Still, as a nation, we get heavier, more sedentary, and less healthy. Until physical activity is viewed as prevention and prevention is viewed as cost effective by the complex of corporations and health care providers, we will continue to travel in the wrong direction on the path of health. Until that time, we are totally on our own. We each have to be responsible for our own health. But that's OK; ultimately we are anyway.

Do you realize that if each of us would say, "I am responsible for my health and I'm going to do something about it," almost all of our country's medical problems and expenses would disappear? The financial structure of the current medical system would collapse. There would be too many healthy people. I know it won't happen. So I have just one realistic wish. I wish you passions and dreams, and I wish one of your passions and one of your dreams would be to make physical activity a part of your life.

Passions and dreams are powerful. I'll share with you two short thoughts on the subject that have helped me. The first is a short poem written by my son:

A dream appears miraculous and startling on our
   horizon;
glowing red, orange, yellow, ignited by an internal sun.
A dream illuminates our future, casting our past into
   shadow,
revealing what we can, what we hope to, what we might
   become.
A dream comforts and inspires and blinds us to
   hardship.
It leads us; a beckoning, twinkling, ethereal beacon,
   through our life.
In the pursuit of our dreams we live.
They are the stuff that life is made of.

The second is a quotation from Dr. Jean-Louis Étienne, who walked alone to the North Pole.

> There are two great times of happiness—when you are haunted by a dream and when you realize it. Between the two there's a strong urge to let it all drop. But you have to follow your dreams to the end. There are abandoned bicycles in every garage because their owner's backsides got too sore the first time they rode them. They don't understand that challenge is a necessary part of learning. I almost gave up a thousand times before reaching those moments of happiness when I forgot that I was cold. You can accomplish this through painting or music or anything, as long as you concede that, before you can play a Bach sonata, you must first learn to play the scales.

I wrote *The 10-Minute L.E.A.P.* to help you learn the scales that can help you make physical activity part of your life. Mr. Millett, a former neighbor and another hero of mine, made physical activity a part of his life. Let me use him as a final example.

I used to live in Farmington, Maine. Every time I drove to or from town I passed Mr. Millett's farm. Mr. Millett never moved fast, but he was usually moving. When I went to school in the morning he was working around the barn. When I came home in the early evening he was still in his fields. Whenever I passed the farm he was busy doing something—not fast, but doing it.

Mr. Millett also had a love of life and an immense curiosity. He became a role model for me. I finally asked him how he could keep on working so consistently. As was his custom, he gave a short answer. He said, "Pace."

One Saturday shortly before noon, I drove past his farm.

He was up on a ladder pruning a tree. When I came back 30 minutes later, he had climbed 10 feet higher in the tree and was sitting in the branches, eating lunch, obviously enjoying the view of his fields.

Mr. Millett was eighty-three.

Perhaps L.E.A.P. will enable you to make physical activity a safe and enjoyable habit. Perhaps, whatever your activity interests and goals, you will gain as much from being physically active as did Mr. Millett.

SOME L.E.A.P. DEFINITIONS

Physical Activity: Physical activity encompasses all physical endeavors, not just exercise. An active lifestyle can include exercise, but is not limited to it. Physical activity creates *challenge*.

Challenge: A challenge is a demand placed upon the *resources* of the body. The level of the challenge presented by a physical activity and perceived by the body/mind depends upon personal characteristics, lifestyle, the type, duration, and intensity of the activity, and the environment where the activity occurs.

Resources: Resources are the systems of the body and the condition of those systems. The systems respond to challenge by converting energy for, among other things, thinking, reacting, providing support, and moving. The result of making physical activity a part of your life is improvement of the systems and an increase in available resources. In order to improve, the systems need *recovery* time.

Recovery: Recovery takes place through the absence of challenge and through the practice of recovery techniques such as supplying proper nutrients at the correct time, getting enough sleep, being able to relax, and when appropriate, using therapeutic modalities to help improve recovery. During recovery, *adaptation* takes place.

Adaptation: Adaptation is the result of improving resources. Adaptation is stimulated by challenge but *only* occurs during recovery. Too much challenge and you will burn out. Too much recovery and you will rust out. The secret to a successful physical activity program is to balance appropriate challenge with sufficient recovery, thereby creating adaptation.

Energy Conversion Number: This number accounts for physical characteristics, lifestyle, and goals that set you apart as an individual. It represents your body's ability to convert energy and correlates with VO_2Max.

VO_2Max : VO_2Max is the maximum volume (V) of oxygen (O_2) you are able to remove from the air, transfer to the blood, deliver to the cells, and use for energy conversion. It is used throughout the L.E.A.P. program to determine Energy Conversion Points and establishes your VO_2Max Coefficient.

VO_2Max Coefficient: The VO_2Max Coefficient is a number representing your VO_2Max and is used to help determine Week 1 Optimal ECPs, your starting point in the L.E.A.P. program. This number modifies your VO_2Max to account for the exponential character of energy conversion as VO_2Max and % VO_2Max change.

Energy Conversion Points (ECPs): ECPs represent the amount of energy converted with each physical activity. By adding ECPs together for the week you can see how close you are to reaching your optimal weekly ECPs goal. ECPs are calculated from your *$VO_2MaxWgtCoef$*, the duration of your activity, and the *Intensity Coefficent*.

$VO_2MaxWgtCoef$: This is a number you use every time you compute ECPs. It simplifies the math because it reduces to three the number of terms you have to deal with. This coefficient is composed of your VO_2Max, body weight, the number of milliliters in a liter, and the number of pounds in a kilogram.

Intensity Coefficient: Intensity coefficients are one of the three numbers used to determine ECPs and are derived from your selection of an intensity level on the Modified Borg–Noble Intensity Scale.

Modified Borg–Noble Intensity Scale: This scale was developed by Dr. Gunnar Borg and Dr. Bruce Noble to help people rate the intensity of effort they perceived when they engaged in physical activity. This rating is referred to as Rating of Perceived Exertion (RPE).

ECPs Formula: The ECPs formula means that by being able to multiply 3 numbers together you have the tool you need to make physical activity a part of your life.

$$ECPs = VO2_{MaxWgtCoef} \times Duration \times I_{Coef}$$

GETTING YOUR L.E.A.P. NUMBERS

*E*arlier you determined your Energy Conversion Number, VO_{2Max}, Week 1 Optimal ECPs, $VO_{2Max}WgtCoef$, 13-week program, and yearly program. This appendix includes all the tables and formulas you need to obtain the same information. If you have any questions you can go back to those chapters and get a full explanation of what the tables mean and how to fill them in.

You may want to copy this appendix so that you can have clean copies of the tables when you want to redo your numbers in the future.

THE AUTOBIOGRAPHY

AGE

Table 19.1

Age	Score
30 or less	4
31 to 40	3
41 to 65	2
Over 65	1

AGE SCORE = _____

GENDER

Enter –1 if pregnant, 0 if not pregnant.

Pregnancy Score _____

FAT-FREE WEIGHT

Step 1. Frame, Leanness, Muscle Bulk/Tone Adjustment.

Table 19.2

Frame	Frame Score	Leanness	Leanness Score	Muscle Bulk	Muscle Score
Very Small	–2	Overweight *or* Too Lean	–4	It's There Somewhere	–3
			-3		–2
Small	–1	Not Lean	–2	Less Than Other People	–1
Average	0	Average	0	Average	0
Large	+1	Lean	+2	More Than Other People	+2
			+3		+3
Very Large	+2	Very Lean	+4	Much More Than Other People	+4
Your Score _____			_____		_____
			ADJUSTMENT SCORE		_____

Body Composition Adjustment

21 + or – adjustment score = _____

Step 2. L.E.A.P. Modified Body Mass Index

$$\frac{Body\ Weight\ (pounds)\ x\ 1130\ (males)\ or\ 1270 (females)}{Height\ (inches)\ x\ Height\ (inches)}$$

EQUATION

Males
____ *(pounds)* x *1130* ÷ ____ *(inches)* x ____ *(inches)=* ____
(to one decimal place)

Females
____ *(pounds)* x *1270* ÷ ____ *(inches)* x ____ *(inches)=* ____
(to one decimal place)

Your Modified Body Mass Index = _____

Step 3. Estimated % Fat Weight
Estimated % Fat Weight = Modified Body Mass Index –
Frame, Leanness, Muscle Bulk Adjustment

_____ - _____ = _____
Your Estimated % Fat Weight = _____

Step 4. Estimated % Fat-Free Weight
Estimated % Fat-Free Weight = 100 – Estimated % Fat Weight
100 - _____ = _____
Your Estimated % Fat-Free Weight = _____

Table 19.3

Level of Fat-Free Weight	% Men	% Women	Fat-Free Weight Score
Usually Too High	≥92	≥88	2.5
Very Healthy	≥86<92	≥82<88	4
Healthy	≥77<86	≥73<82	3
Could Be Higher	≥70<77	≥66<73	2
Too Low	<70	<66	1

Fat-Free Weight Score

Your Fat-Free Weight Score = _____

SLEEP

Table 19.4

Question	Usually	Sometimes	Not Usually	Score
Do you drink beverages with caffeine or alcohol within 3 hours of going to bed?	1	2	3	_____
Do you have a relaxing routine before going to bed?	3	2	1	_____
Do you go to bed about the same time each night?	4	2	1	_____
Is there fresh air in your bedroom?	3	2	1	_____
Is your bedroom dark and quiet?	3	2	1	_____
Is your sleeping surface too hard/too soft?	1	2	3	_____
Do you have trouble getting to sleep?	1	2	4	_____
If you wake up during the night, do you have trouble getting back to sleep?	1	2	3	_____
Do you get up about the same time, even on weekends?	4	2	1	_____
Do you get up naturally, without an alarm?	3	2	1	_____
Are you still tired when you get up?	1	2	3	_____
Do you get the amount of sleep you feel you need?	4	2	0	_____
			Total	_____
		Total ÷ 12		_____

Sleep Score

In the Sleep segment, round off to two decimal places.

Your Sleep Score = _____

RELAXATION

Table 19.5

Question	Not Usually	Sometimes	Usually	Score
Do you have headaches?	3	2	1	_____
Do you easily get angry?	3	2	1	_____
Do you easily get anxious?	3	2	1	_____
Is it difficult for you to concentrate?	3	2	1	_____
Is it easy for you to laugh?	1	2	3	_____
Do coworkers think you are in a good mood?	1	2	3	_____
Do you feel energetic?	1	2	3	_____
Do you practice relaxation techniques or do *easy* aerobic exercises?	1	2	4	_____
			Total	_____
			Total ÷ 8	_____

Relaxation Score

In the Relaxation segment, round off to two decimal places.

Your Relaxation Score = _____

NUTRITION

Table 19.6

Question	Usually	Sometimes	Not Usually	Score
Do you eat fresh vegetables each day?	4	2	1	_____
Do you eat fresh fruit each day?	4	2	1	_____
Do you eat some legumes (beans, seeds, or sprouts) each day?	3	2	1	_____
Do you eat nutritious grains each day?	3	2	1	_____
If you are not allergic, do you consume some, but not too many, dairy products each day? If allergic, do you get calcium from another source?	3	2	1	_____
Do you eat some meat, but not too much, or get protein from another source, each day?	3	2	1	_____
Do you try to buy organic/ chemical-free food?	3	2	1	_____
Are labels important in selecting what you eat?	3	2	1	_____
Do you try to buy mostly fresh foods as opposed to processed?	3	2	1	_____
In preparing foods, do you try to maintain nutritional value and minimize detrimental ingredients?	3	2	1	_____
Do you try to minimize fast food?	3	2	1	_____
Do you try to minimize junk food?	3	2	1	_____
Do you try minimize caffeine-based drinks?	3	2	1	_____
Are you a moderate or nondrinker?	Yes = 3	1	−2	_____
Are you a nonsmoker?	Yes = 3	0	−3	_____
			Total	_____
			Total ÷ 15	_____

Nutrition Score

In the Nutrition segment, round off to two decimal places.

Your Nutrition Score = _____

CURRENT PHYSICAL ACTIVITY

Table 19.7

Value	Category	Days/Week	Minutes/Day	Intensity (%VO2Max)	Value
6	National/World-Class Competitor	7	> 90	85 Strong+	6
5.5	College Competitor	6	75-90	80	5.5
5	Adult Competitor	5	60-75	75	5
4.5	Active Adult	4	50-60	70	4.5
4	HS Competitor	3	40-50	65 Somewhat Strong	4
3.5	Age Group Competitor	2	30-40	60	3.5
3	Somewhat Active Young Adult	1	20-30	55 Moderate	3
2.5	Somewhat Active Student	Seasonal + Sporadic	15–20	50	2.5
2	Somewhat Active Adult	Better Than Sporadic	10-15	45 Easy	2
1.5	In Rehab	Sporadic	1-10	40 Very Easy	1.5
1	Inactive	Inactive	0	Nothing At All	1
	Category Score ___	Day/Week Score ___	Minute Score ___	Intensity Score ___	

Total Score _____
Total Score ÷ 4 _____

Current Physical Activity

In the Current Physical Activity segment, round off to two decimal places.

Your Current Physical Activity Score = _____

ENERGY CONVERSION NUMBER

Table 19.8

Segment	Score
Age Score	_____
Pregnancy Score (if applicable)	_____
Fat-Free Weight Score	_____
Sleep Score	_____
Relaxation Score	_____
Nutrition Score	_____
Current Physical Activity Score	_____
Total	_____

Energy Conversion Number

Your Energy Conversion Number = _____

VO2MAX

Find the Energy Conversion Number that is closest to yours. In the column to the right of that number is your VO2Max.

Table 19.9

Conversion Number	VO2Max	Conversion Number	VO2Max	Conversion Number	VO2Max
23.51	72	18.92	49	9.30	26
23.39	71	18.59	48	8.97	25
23.28	70	18.26	47	8.64	24
23.16	69	17.93	46	8.31	23
23.05	68	17.46	45	7.98	22
22.93	67	17.00	44	7.66	21
22.82	66	16.53	43	7.33	20
22.70	65	16.06	42	7.00	19
22.58	64	15.60	41	6.67	18
22.47	63	15.13	40	6.34	17
22.35	62	14.66	39	6.02	16
22.24	61	14.19	38	5.69	15
22.12	60	13.73	37	5.36	14
22.01	59	13.26	36		
21.89	58	12.80	35		
21.56	57	12.33	34		
21.23	56	11.87	33		
20.90	55	11.40	32		
20.57	54	10.94	31		
20.24	53	10.61	30		
19.91	52	10.28	29		
19.58	51	9.95	28		
19.25	50	9.62	27		

Energy Conversion Number and VO2Max

Your VO2Max = _____ ml/kg/min

WEEK 1 OPTIMAL ECPS

SUPPORT AND TIME

Table 19.10

Question	Usually	Sometimes	Not Usually	Score
Do you make physical activity as important as any other item on your calendar?	4	2	1	_____
Does your partner share or support your physical activity? (2 if not applicable)	4	2	1	_____
Do your family/friends share or support your physical activity?	3	2	1	_____
Does your employer support your physical activity? (2 if not applicable)	3	2	1	_____
Do you work 40 hours per week or less?	3	2	1	_____
Do you spend less than 4 hours a week on other obligations, such as school, church, clubs?	3	2	1	_____
If you live with children, does it help make you more physically active? (3 if not applicable)	3	2	1	_____
Do you watch less than 10 hours of TV/videos a week?	3	2	1	_____
			Total	_____
			Total ÷ 8	_____

Support/Time Score

Your Support/Time Score = _____

WEEK 1 COEFFICENT

Table 19.11

Activity Category	Week 1 Coefficient
National/WC Competitor	.141
College Competitor	.116
Adult Competitor	.082
HS Competitor	.057
Active Adult	.047
Age group Competitor	.032
Somewhat Active Young Adult	.023
Somewhat Active Student	.019
Somewhat Active Adult	.017
In Rehabilitation	.009
Inactive	.004

Week 1 Coefficent

Your Week 1 Coefficent= _____

VO₂MAX COEFFICENT

Table 19.12

VO₂Max	VO₂Max< Coef	VO₂Max	VO₂Max Coef	VO₂Max	VO₂Max Coef
72	42.86	52	26.51	32	12.94
71	41.99	51	25.76	31	12.35
70	41.12	50	25.01	30	11.76
69	40.25	49	24.28	29	11.19
68	39.39	48	23.55	28	10.62
67	38.54	47	22.83	27	10.07
66	37.69	46	22.12	26	9.52
65	36.85	45	21.41	25	8.99
64	36.02	44	20.71	24	8.46
63	35.19	43	20.02	23	7.94
62	34.37	42	19.33	22	7.44
61	33.55	41	18.66	21	6.95
60	32.74	40	17.99	20	6.46
59	31.94	39	17.33	19	5.99
58	31.15	38	16.68	18	5.53
57	30.36	37	16.03	17	5.08
56	29.57	36	15.40	16	4.65
55	28.80	35	14.77	15	4.23
54	28.03	34	14.15	14	3.82
53	27.26	33	13.54		

VO₂Max Coefficent

Your VO₂Max Coefficient = _____

YOUR WEEK 1 OPTIMAL ECPS

Step 1.   *Your Week 1 Coef =* _____
Your Vo2MaxCoef = _____
Your Support/Time Score = _____
Your Weight = _____

Step 2. *Multiply those four values.*

Step 3. *Your Week 1 Optimal ECPs =* _____ *ECPs or Liters O2/wk*

VO2MAXWgtCoef

Your VO2MaxCoef = _____
Your Weight = _____

VO2MaxWgtCoef = VO2MaxCoef x Weight/1936

_____ x _____ /1936 = _____

LEVELS

Level = VO2MaxWgtCoef x Frequency x Duration x ICoef

Safe Minimum = _____ x 7 x 10 x .26   = _____

Risk Reduction = _____ x 7 x 30 x .37   = _____

Body Change = _____ x 4 x 30 x .82   = _____

VO2Max Change = _____ x 4 x 40 x .82   = _____

Optimal = *Week 1 Optimal ECPs* = _____

Overtraining = *Optimal x 1.075* = _____

ZONES

Success $\geq$ *Risk Reduction* $\geq$ _____

Optimal $\geq$ *Optimal x .925* $\geq$ _____

Overtraining $>$ *Optimal x 1.075* $>$ _____

	Success Zone	**Optimal Zone**	**Overtraining Zone**
Safe Minimum = _____			

First fill in the beginning of your success zone, then the beginning of the optimal zone, and then the beginning of the overtraining zone.

Second, fill in the levels (risk reduction, body change, VO2Max change, and optimal) in the zone in which they fit as shown in the earlier examples.

13-WEEK MAINTENANCE PROGRAM

In a Maintenance Program, you do not increase ECPs each week. The table allows you to put in ECPs for each of the 13 weeks. Just put your Week 1 ECPs in the first 10 weeks. In Week 11 put in 75% of the Week 1 ECPs, and in Week 12 put in 50% of the Week 1 ECPs. Week 13 is the rest week.

Table 19.13

Week #	Cycle #1
1	
2	
3	
4	
5	
6	
7	
8	
9	
10	
11	
12	
13	0

13-Week Maintenance Program

13-WEEK PROGRESSION PROGRAM

Find the Energy Conversion Number that is closest to yours. Then read across the line to get the % Increase you will use.

%INCREASE

Table 19.14

VO2Max	% Increase	VO2Max	%Increase	VO2Max	% Increase
72	.0018	52	.0086	31	.0141
71	.0021	51	.0088	30	.0143
70	.0023	50	.0091	29	.0146
69	.0028	49	.0093	28	.0148
68	.0031	48	.0098	27	.0151
67	.0033	47	.0101	26	.0153
66	.0036	46	.0103	25	.0156
65	.0038	45	.0106	24	.0158
64	.0043	44	.0108	23	.0161
63	.0046	43	.0111	22	.0163
62	.0048	42	.0113	21	.0166
61	.0051	41	.0116	20	.0168
60	.0053	40	.0118	19	.0171
59	.0056	39	.0121	18	.0173
58	.0061	38	.0123	17	.0176
56	.0073	37	.0126	16	.0178
57	.0068	36	.0218	15	.0181
55	.0076	35	.0131	14	.0183
54	.0078	34	.0133		
53	.0081	33	.0136		
		32	.0138		

% Increase

Your % Increase = _____

13-WEEK PROGRESSION

Step 1. Your Week 1 Optimal ECPs = _____

Step 2. Your % Increase = _____

Step 3. Your ECPs Increase = Week 1 ECPs x % Increase = _____ (round off to whole number)

Step 4. Fill in the table following according to following instructions:

1. Week 1: Enter your Week 1 ECPs.
2. Week 2: Enter the sum of your Week 1 Optimal ECPs plus your ECPs Increase.
3. Week 3: Enter the sum of Week 2 plus your ECPs Increase.
4. Weeks 4 through 10: Repeat by adding the previous week to the ECPs Increase.
5. Week 11: Enter the ECPs from Week 3.
6. Week 12: Subtract two (2) times the ECPs Increase from Week 1 Optimal ECPs.
7. Week 13: A recovery week; 0 points has already been entered.

Table 19.15

Week #	Cycle #1
1	
2	
3	
4	
5	
6	
7	
8	
9	
10	
11	
12	
13	0

13-Week Progression Program

SETTING UP A 1-YEAR PROGRAM

If you want a full year's Maintenance Program, all you need to do is fill in the table by repeating the cycle for the first 13-week Maintenance Program.

If you want a full year's Progression Program, repeat the instructions for Cycle 1 to obtain Cycles 2, 3, and 4. Week 1 ECPs will be the optimal ECPs from Week 5 of the preceding cycle.

Table 19.16

Week	Cycle 1	Cycle 2	Cycle 3	Cycle 4
1	_____	_____	_____	_____
2	_____	_____	_____	_____
3	_____	_____	_____	_____
4	_____	_____	_____	_____
5	_____	_____	_____	_____
6	_____	_____	_____	_____
7	_____	_____	_____	_____
8	_____	_____	_____	_____
9	_____	_____	_____	_____
10	_____	_____	_____	_____
11	_____	_____	_____	_____
12	_____	_____	_____	_____
13	0	0	0	0

1-Year Program

SUGGESTED DAILY PERCENTAGE
OF WEEKLY ECPS

Table 19.17

Days/ Week Active	Day 1	Day 2	Day 3	Day 4	Day 5	Day 6	Day 7
3	33		33		33		
4	30		22		26		22
5	26	12	20		22		20
6	24	12	16		20	12	16
7	22	10	15	10	18	10	15

Daily Percentages of Weekly ECPs

The maximum you should ever do on any one day is 40% of your optimal ECPs.

L.E.A.P. LOGS

Each time you are active, you figure how much energy you converted by that activity:

Daily ECPs = VO2MaxWgtCoef x Duration x Icoef

You can then enter this information in the L.E.A.P. Weekly Log and add these to your weekly total and compare them with your weekly goal.

Table 19.18

Date _____ VO2Max _____ Success Optimal Optimal Overtng 40% Risk Reduction = _____
Cycle _____ WgtCoef= _____ Zone ≥ _____ Zone ≥ _____ Level = _____ Zone> _____ ECPs = _____ Body Change = _____
Week _____ VO2MaxChange = _____

Day	Activities	Duration (min)	ICoef	ECPs (Act)	Total ECPs (day)	Total (wk)	ECPs Left	Comments
1								
2								
3								
4								
5								
6								
7								
Totals		Total Time	ECPs /Min			Total ECPs		

Zone (Circle 1)   Success/Optimal/OT

Sample L.E.A.P. Weekly Log

Table 19.19

Cycle # Week #	Duration	ECPs	ECPs/ Min	Success Zone	Optimal Zone	Overtng Zone	Calories= (ECPsx4.85)	Pounds Not Gained= (Cal÷3500)
1								
2								
3								
4								
5								
6								
7								
8								
9								
10								
11								
12								
13								
Totals								

L.E.A.P. 13-Week Log

HOW TO ESTIMATE YOUR INTENSITY

*E*stimating intensity by perceived exertion can be done by almost everyone. The technique was developed by Dr. Gunnar Borg in the late 1960s. Dr. Borg believed perceived exertion to be the single best indicator of the degree of physical strain because it integrates information from the working muscles and joints, from the cardiovascular and respiratory systems, and from the central nervous system.

According to Dr. Michael Pollock, who has worked extensively with perceived exertion, "even though the scale is psychological, it has a lot of physiological meaning," the perceptions of difficulty correlate well with measurements of pulse, oxygen consumption, lactic acid production, and breathing.

L.E.A.P. uses a Borg-Noble Intensity Scale that has been expanded to include %VO2Max, depth and rate of breathing, and ability to talk. There are four basic instructions to observe when using the Modified Borg-Noble Intensity Scale. The first three are quoted from Dr. Borg:

1. During exercise, rate your perception of exertion.

2. Rate that feeling as honestly as possible. Some people want to be "brave" and rate too low. Try your best to rate your exertion as you perceive it.

3. Don't consider the exercise goal or the size of the task. The only thing of interest is your own feeling of effort and exertion.

4. If you are doing an intermittent activity, average the overall intensity of the session.

The Modified Borg-Noble Intensity Scale also shows how %VO2Max coincides with a shift in the physiological responses of the body.

55% VO2Max—Start of a pronounced benefit from physical activity

65% VO2Max—Sense that you are putting forth some effort

75% VO2Max—In a zone where you could continue for a long time if you had to, but effort is getting strong

85% VO2Max—Sense that if you worked much harder, the rate of physiological functions would sharply increase; somewhere near the edge of steady state work

90% VO2Max—In a zone where your body has to work very hard to keep the environment of the cell stable

Table 20.1

RPE	Challenge was	Breathing was	Talking was	%VO2Max	ICoef
1.0	Very Easy	Normal	Normal	35	**0.08**
1.5				40	**0.16**
2.0	Easy	Normal	Normal	45	**0.26**
2.5				50	**0.37**
3.0	Moderate	Comfortable	Easy	55	**0.51**
3.5				60	**0.66**
4.0	Somewhat Strong	Noticeable	Somewhat Difficult	65	**0.82**
4.5				70	**1.00**
5.0	Strong	Deep, but Steady	Difficult	75	**1.20**
5.5				80	**1.40**
6.0	Between Strong & Very Strong	Deep & Somewhat Rapid	Between Difficult & Very Difficult	85	**1.62**
6.5				87.5	**1.86**
7.0	Very Strong	Deep & Rapid	Very Difficult	90	**2.10**
7.5				92.5	**2.36**
8.0	Very, Very Strong	Very Deep & Very Rapid	Extremely Difficult	95	**2.63**
8.5				96.1	**2.91**
9.0				97.5	**3.21**
9.5				98.8	**3.51**
10	Maximum Effort	Breathlessness	Impossible	100	**3.83**

Modified Borg-Noble Intensity Scale

When using this scale it is all right to interpolate between the listed intensity coefficients.

*U*sing heart rate to measure intensity is valid if done correctly. There are two ways to do it. One is to take your heart rate (pulse rate) manually immediately after you finish exercise and use that as an indication of how hard you were working. Like the muscle-to-fat ratio, it will be a relative measurement and can help fix your intensity compared with other physical activity sessions you have done. Of course, if you do intermittent exercise you will have to average, just as with RPE.

You shouldn't compare your heart rate with charts or formulas that say they can tell you what your rate should be based on age. We are all individuals. The athletes I coach are near the same age but all have different maximum and resting heart rates. Using formulas like (220 – Age) or (210 – (.65 x Age)) may not be accurate for you. Table 21.1 shows the differences in these two formulas:

Table 21.1

Age	220-Age	210-(.65 x Age)
30	190	191
40	180	184
50	170	178
60	160	171
70	150	165

Heart Rate Formula Comparisons

When you are dealing with heart rate you want to be as accurate as possible. It appears to be an objective measurement, but without a measured maximum heart rate it is just a guess. If you work out at too low a percentage of your maximum heart rate, providing you know what that is, you will not get the results you want. Much more dangerous is working out at too high a percentage. At that range you risk overtraining and injury.

If you want to use your heart rate to train and don't have a heart rate monitor, you should be aware of the fact that the heart rate can drop as much as 10% to 20% in a few seconds depending upon how hard you are exercising. I coach an athlete who because of heart surgery monitors her heart rate both manually and with a heart rate monitor. We did a little experiment. I asked her to look at her monitor as soon as she stopped running and then immediately take her pulse manually. Her heart rate on the monitor as soon as she stopped was 142; by the time she had taken a 15-second pulse count it was down to 130. We repeated this frequently, always with the same results.

Taking the usual 10-second count may not be enough to eliminate this decline, but if you take a 6-second count you introduce an error because in 6 seconds you could easily miss or add a beat on each end of the count. Then when you multiply by 10 to get your beats per minute, you could be off by as many as 20 beats. Still, the 6-second count is probably the best way to measure without a heart rate monitor if, instead of multiplying the result by another number, you regard the result directly. This method will give you relative information with respect to the intensity of each workout. For example, if you got a 15 for the count after one workout and a 13 after another, you know the first workout was probably done at a higher intensity.

The absolute best way to use heart rate is to follow these instructions.

1. Purchase a reliable heart rate monitor. I have found that Polar heart rate monitors (1-800-227-1314) are reliable and offer a variety of features.
2. Get a valid maximum heart rate from a professional. This will involve a maximum effort and must be done in a proper testing environment.
3. Determine your resting heart rate. You can do this by taking your morning heart rate for 10 to 14 days and averaging the results. You should take the heart rate before you get out of bed by counting your pulse for 60 seconds.
4. Determine your heart rate reserve.

Heart Rate Reserve = Heart Rate$_{Max}$ − Heart Rate$_{Rest}$

5. It turns out that %VO$_2$Max is close to %Heart Rate Reserve. If you want to work out at a specific %VO$_2$Max and you are using a heart rate monitor, you can figure out what your heart rate should be. Just multiply the %VO$_2$Max by the heart rate reserve and add the resting heart rate. The number is the heart rate at which you should work out.

EXAMPLE

My Heart Rate$_{Max}$ = 178
My Heart Rate$_{Rest}$ = 51
My Heart Rate$_{Reserve}$ = 127

I want to work out at 75% VO$_2$Max.
Exercise Heart Rate = (127 x .75) + 51 = 146
I should work out at about 146 beats per minute.

L.E.A.P. ACTIVITY LIST

*T*hese are not the only activities you can do to convert energy. This is just a list that may help give you some ideas. In reality you are limited only by your imagination. When you use L.E.A.P. and %VO2Max for estimation of intensity, any physical activity that converts energy counts.

L.E.A.P. ACTIVITY LIST
Adventure/Outdoor

Backpacking
Bongee Jumping
Diving
   Board
   Scuba
   Skin
   Sky
Fishing
   Bank
   Boat
   Ocean
   Wade
Hiking
Horseback Riding
Hunting
Mountain Biking
Parachuting

Rock Climbing
Skating
   Board
   Ice
   In-Line
Skiing
   Downhill
   Roller
   Water
Snorkeling
Snowboarding
Snowshoeing
Surfing
   Board
   Body
   Wind

Aerobics

Aerobics
Run-in-Water
  Bottom
  Deep
Slide Aerobics
Step Aerobics

Tread Water
Water Aerobics
  Deep
  Shallow

Combatant Sports

Boxing
Fencing
Judo

Karate
Wrestling
Other Martial Arts

Dance

Ballet
Ballroom
Contemporary

Modern
Tap

Distance/Pace Activities

Bicycling
Cross-Country Skiing
Jogging or Running
Jogging and Walking
Racewalking
Swimming
Treadmill

Walking
  Heavy Hands
  Normal
  Rapid
Wheelchair Push

Exercise Equipment/Machines

Airdyne-type Machine
Bicycle
  Recumbent Stationary
  Spinning
  Upright Stationary
Concept II–type Rowing Machine
Healthrider–type Machine
Jump Rope
Nordic Track–type Skiing Machine
Stair Climbing
Stair Master–type Machine
Trampoline
  Mini
  Regular
VersaClimber–type Machine

Games/Sports

Archery
Badminton
Baseball
Basketball
Billiards
Bowling
Croquet
Football
  Tackle
  Touch
Frisbee
Golf
  Cart
  Driving Range
  Walk
Gymnastics
Handball
Hockey
  Field
  Ice
  Street

Horseshoes
Lacrosse
Paddleball
Racquetball
Rugby
Shooting
Shuffleboard
Soccer
Softball
Squash
Table Tennis
Tennis
  Singles
  Doubles
Volleyball
  Court
  Sand
Wallyball

Home/Work Activities

Bed Rehabilitation Exercises
Gardening
Housework

Manual Labor
Rehabilitation Exercises
Sexual Activity

Strength/Flexibility Training

Body Building
Calisthenics
Circuit Training
Stretching

Weight Training
  Endurance
  Power
  Strength
  Tone
Yoga

Water Craft

Canoeing
Jet Boating
Kayaking
Rafting
Rowing
  Boat
  Shell

Sail Boarding
Sailing
  Lake
  Ocean

You already know some of the things you should be doing with your diet from the discussion of nutrition in the Autobiography section. Let me share with you how I confront the issue of nutrition in my own day-to-day life and what I suggest to the athletes I coach.

For over 25 years my daughter and I have more or less followed what we informally call the "The Big Day Diet." All that means is that for 6 days of the week we eat intelligently and on the 7th we eat whatever we want and as much of it as we want–the Big Day! We figured we could stick to anything for 6 days as long as we had some freedom to choose whatever we craved at the end of that short tunnel. The discipline of the first 6 days makes you feel good about yourself, and the Big Day is a way to reward yourself on the 7th. The whole plan is enjoyable. The diet is nutritious. And we both noticed a funny thing–after awhile your body doesn't crave a Big Day anymore, and many of them pass without you even knowing they've arrived. Here are the simple rules of the Big Day Diet.

BIG DAY DIET CONCEPT 1—EAT BREAKFAST

Eating a nutritious breakfast does your body a big favor. Your body has been on a short 8- to 10-hour fast during which time it was rebuilding. You are now becoming more active and require additional energy. If you don't get food into your body soon after you wake up, the body will start to use glucose reserves, which further depletes your energy stores. The body also perceives that food is not available and will tend to conserve fat for a "rainy day."

By not eating a decent breakfast you deplete energy stores, convert some protein (muscle) into energy, and conserve fat. In fact, prisoners released from concentration camps still had some fat reserves. The reason they were so thin is that they had used most of their muscle tissue for fuel while their bodies conserved their fat as a final resource in the face of starvation.

A fast food or junk food breakfast is not a nutritious breakfast, and it often results in a sugar high. This upsets your body's balance, stimulating an insulin response, which removes blood sugar. Then you are faced with a sugar low. This cycle can often repeat itself throughout the day, resulting in the ingestion of more sugar than you can convert to work or heat. So the energy is stored as fat.

A junk food or fast food breakfast can also give you a fat high, which may even be worse. Fat is used in foods to enhance taste because saturated fat tastes good. But it is a dangerous type of fat, and what the body does with it is store it in arteries or fat cells.

Avoid caffeine too. Caffeine gives you a boost by releasing adrenaline. But this is like stimulating the "fight or flight" mechanism and further depletes energy reserves, with the added burden of wasting adrenaline and keying up the body with no physical outlet in sight.

BIG DAY DIET CONCEPT 2—EAT THE RIGHT FOODS IN THE RIGHT AMOUNTS

Each day when you get up you should subconsciously understand that before the day is over you will provide your body with the energy and nutrients it needs. You should have it in your mind that part of the day is devoted to making sure you fulfill your nutritional needs. This raises the question: What type of food and how much of it fulfills your nutritional needs?

First, what. Foods are carriers for calories and nutrients. The nutrients you need to take into your body are carbohydrates, proteins, fats, minerals, vitamins, and fiber. Very few people can keep track of what nutrients are in the foods they eat, much less know how much of each is in everything. If they try to record the nutrients and their amounts, they soon stop, exhausted and frustrated. It's best simply to know what foods to eat.

Foods are commonly divided into groups. Since the body requires food from each of the food groups, you shouldn't think that you can compensate for consistently missing one food group by eating more from another food group. Each food group provides its own essential nutrients.

Six years ago I found a book that does an excellent job of discussing proper nutrition. Dr. Roy Vartebadian took a major step toward simplifying the problem when he wrote the book *NutriPoints*. In it he evaluated the nutrients in all the foods you'd ever want to eat and gave a point value to each food. His ratings eliminated the need to examine the foods for all their different nutrients and substituted an overall point value that accounted for the ingredients.

I have modified Dr. Vartebadian's system by giving the top scorers in each food group a 10-point value and by making serving sizes equal. This makes it easier to see the relative worth of the foods within each group. Remember, don't compare foods from different groups, because we need food from each of the six groups. Some of the foods with their modified scores are listed in the table at the end of this appendix.This is by no means a complete listing, but instead is included to provide some basis for comparison.

In the *NutriPoints* system, foods receive either a positive or a negative score. Foods that receive a positive score help you effectively replenish your resources and live a healthy life. Many foods that receive a negative score detract from your overall ability to replenish energy and rebuild resources. The calories you get by eating these foods may be termed *questionable calories.* Because they do not provide the nutrients required for their processing, they often take more from the body's resources than they give, or they add things the body does not need. They can be looked at as nutrient-free calories and are often expensive foods with respect to performance, health, and dollars. That doesn't mean you can't eat these foods. It just means that they should not be looked upon as substitutes for real food and that their intake should be limited.

Now, the how much. Forget measuring in cups, tablespoons, and ounces. Measure in easily managed handfuls. How much of the food can you easily hold in one hand? The handful works well in a practical sense because it is a readily available measuring device and estimates of handfuls are easily understood. A handful usually equals a cup. Also, an assumption can be made that bigger (not fatter) people require more food, and this will usually be provided for by their larger hands.

Using the handful system doesn't mean you have to scoop food up in your hand. You usually just have to estimate what a handful looks like. The table below shows the food groups and the suggested handfuls of each food group per day for a person with about 130 pounds of fat-free body weight. It also shows how to adjust the serving sizes based on pounds of fat-free body weight. For example, if you have 30 more pounds of fat-free weight (160 pounds), you might add two servings of water, a couple of more servings of vegetables, and another serving of fruits and grains. If you had 30 less pounds of fat-free weight (100 pounds) you would subtract the same amount.

Table 23.1

Food Group	Handsful per 130 pounds of Fat-Free Weight	Add or Subtract One Handful per Listed Pounds of Fat-Free Weight
Water	6–10	15
Vegetables	6–7	20
Fruits	4–5	30
Grains	3–4	40
Milk/Dairy	2–3	50
Legumes	1–2	90
Meat/Fish/Poultry	1–2	90
Junk Food/Fast Food	0–2	90

Food Groups and Suggested Servings Per Day

The advantage of eating the right amount from each group is that you automatically get the proper balance of calories, carbohydrates, proteins, fats, minerals, vitamins, and fiber. You don't have to concern yourself with counting all these different nutrients.

You probably noticed water listed as the first ingredient. Getting enough water is crucial. It is the environment in which all your cells must live. If you are short of water, your cells live in an increasingly alien environment.

Eating some negative foods each day is OK. If you are extremely active, know that you will get a proper diet by the end of the day, and you still feel hungry during the day, it's OK to eat foods that have a high caloric content such as cookies. But don't eat junk foods as a substitute for positive foods. Eat them in addition to positive foods when you feel hungry and know that you will be getting all your positive food by the end of the day.

BIG DAY DIET CONCEPT 3—TRY TO EAT AS CLOSE TO NATURE AS POSSIBLE

When you shop for or prepare your food, you should remember that the food value is changed by how the food is grown, processed, and prepared.

Buying food that is certified organic is better than having it merely pesticide-free. Both are preferable to food grown or raised on large commercial farms where heavy chemical use is normal. Your body has to deal with these chemicals by metabolizing them or storing them, a poor use of your body's resources that is sometimes downright dangerous.

Fresh food is better than frozen, which is better than canned, which is better than fully processed. Each step removes food further from its natural state and removes or alters some of the nutrients. Processed food means food that, for example, has been precooked, candied, pickled, or had ingredients added to preserve shelf life, to make it easier to cook, to make it look better, or to enhance flavor.

In food preparation, the order of desirability in most cases is fresh, steamed, boiled, baked, broiled, and, last, fried. Again, the fresher it is, the more nutrients it has retained.

BIG DAY DIET CONCEPT 4—DOLLARS PER NUTRIENT, NOT DOLLARS PER POUND

People say organic food is more expensive. This is usually true if you think in terms of dollars per pound, as we are conditioned to think. Break the mold! Dollar-per-pound thinking is a very expensive way to eat because usually foods that can be sold inexpensively have been processed or handled by large commercial firms that must try to preserve shelf life. This requires removing certain ingredients natural to the food and adding ingredients that make them look attractive, "taste great," or preserve shelf life. These foods have been processed or altered in some way that makes them easier on the pocketbook, easier to prepare, or tempting to the taste. Often this means adding sugar or salt. You may spend less money on this food, but chances are very good that you will eventually spend whatever you save on future health care. It is much better to think in terms of dollars per nutrient. If you buy foods that are as close to natural as possible, you may pay more dollars, but you will get more nutrients.

You may spend more money up front on excellent foods, but you will be eating well. You might even eat a little less because you are getting more nutrients per pound of food. Eating less could provide the added benefit of helping to control weight. Eating the dollar-per-nutrient way will probably add healthy years to your life.

Table 23.1

MODIFIED NUTRIPOINT FOOD LIST

VEGETABLES Plus Foods	FRUITS Plus Foods	GRAINS Plus Foods	LEGUMES/ NUTS/SEEDS Plus Foods
10 brussel sprouts	10 kiwi	10 wheat bran	10 sunflower seeds
8 carrots	9 cantaloupe	8 wheat germ	9 kidney beans
7 spinach	8 blackberries	5 mueslix	9 garbanzo beans
7 broccoli	7 raspberries	5 shredded wheat	9 navy beans
6 asparagus	6 apricots	2 oatmeal	8 peas
5 cauliflower	6 figs	2 familia	8 lima beans
5 cabbage	6 strawberries	2 wild rice	7 pinto beans
4 mushrooms	5 prunes	2 whole wheat noodles	7 roasted pumpkin seeds
4 squash	5 dates	2 brown rice	6 roasted squash seeds
4 pepper	5 pineapple	2 whole grain spaghetti	6 roasted soybeans
3 green beans	5 raisins	1 whole grain macaroni	6 tofu

3 sweet potatoes	4 bananas	1 spanish noodles	6 bean sprouts
3 beets	4 blueberries	1 whole grain bread	5 soybeans
3 cucumbers	4 honeydew melon	1 English muffin	4 lentils
2 potatoes	4 oranges	1 whole grain pancakes	4 baked beans
2 lettuce	4 tangerines	1 white rice	3 dry roasted peanuts
2 celery	4 tomatoes	1 whole grain lasagna	3 unsalted peanutbutter
	4 avacados	1 minute rice	
	4 grapefruit	1 bagel	
	3 sweet cherries	1 whole grain crackers	
	3 peaches	1 whole grain linguine	
	3 watermelon	1 veggie pizza	
	3 cranberries		
	3 nectarines		
	3 plums		
	2 apples		
	2 grapes		
	2 pears		

Neutral Foods	**Neutral Foods**	**Neutral Foods**	**Neutral Foods**
0 pickles	0 cnd fruit, lgt syrp	0 ravioli	0 refried beans
0 fastfood baked potato	0 jello, sugar-free	0 macaroni & cheese	0 regular peanutbutter
0 fastfood taco salad	0 cranberry juice	0 macaroni salad	0 dry roasted cashews
0 instant potatos		0 blueberry muffin	0 honey roasted peanuts
		0 regular mix pancakes	0 frozen bean burritos

Negative Foods	**Negative Foods**	**Negative Foods**	**Negative Foods**
-1 fried onion rings	-.3 cnd fruit, hvy syrp	-.2 banana bread	-2 oil roasted pecans
-1 potato chips	-.3 applesauce w/sugar	-.4 homemade cookies	-2 fastfood tacos
-1 soups, many cmrcl	-1 fruit pies	-.4 granola bars	-3 covered peanuts

-1 french fried potatos

-1 hash brown potatos

-2 fruit drinks

-2 orange sherbet

-2 carob covered rasins

-3 choc covered raisins

-5 jams

-.4 fast food pancakes

-1 fastfood bisquits

-1 croissant

-1 cmrcl fig newton

-1 fastfood french toast

-1 combo/meat pizza

-1 rice pudding

-1 cakes/brownie

-1 fastfood/cmrcl cookies

-1 pastry/dounut/twinkies

-2 fastfood pastry

-4 peanut butter cup

-8 candy bar w/peanuts

-10 peanut brittle

MILK/DIARY	MEATS	CONDIMENTS	MISCELLA NEOUS
Plus Foods	**Plus Foods**	**Plus Foods**	**Plus Foods**
10 non-fat dry milk	10 tuna	10 chili powder	10 brewer's yeast
2 skim milk	9 beef liver, fried, organic	10 paprika	6 protein powder
2 lo-fat cottage cheese	8 salmon	9 green hot chili pepper	6 soy drink
2 non-fat yogurt	8 swordfish	6 red/cayenne pepper	3 carob powder
2 Ovaltine cocoa mix	8 liverwurst, organic	5 picante sauce	1 cocoa powder
2 1% mikl	7 halibut	4 basil	1 consomme
2 2% milk	6 trout	4 lo-salt chckn bouillon	1 sugar-free Kool Ade
2 egg	5 turkey w/o skin	4 celery seed	1 herb tea
1 yogurt dressing	5 chicken w/o skin	4 chives	
	5 baked lean ham	4 cinnamon	
	4 beef	4 ginger	
	4 flounder	4 lemon juice	
	4 red snapper	4 black pepper	
	4 ocean perch	4 poppy seed	

4 sole	4 chili sauce		
3 clam chowder	1 lime juice		
3 scallops	1 raw garlic		
2 haddock	1 lo-salt ketchup		
	1 dried parsley		

Neutral Foods	**Neutral Foods**	**Neutral Foods**	**Neutral Foods**
0 cheddar cheese	0 Canadian bacon	0 equal	0 mineral water
0 grilled cheese sand	0 corned beef	0 vinegar	0 club soda
0 strawberry sundae	0 organic pot pie	0 vanilla extract	0 decaffeinated coffee
0 banana pudding	0 short ribs	0 mustard	
0 frozen yogurt	0 chicken chow mein	0 horseradish	
0 hot chocolate		0 soy sauce	

Negative Foods	**Negative Foods**	**Negative Foods**	**Negative Foods**
-.2 chocolate milk	-1 commercial pot pie	-1 chicken bouillon	-1 flavored water
-1 ice cream	-1 fastfood hamburger	-1 teriyaki sauce	-1 sugar-free ice tea mix
-1 milkshake	-1 fried pork chop	-3 sweet & sour sauce	-2 caffeinated coffee
-1 most cheese	-2 bratwurst	-3 barbecue sauce	
-1 lo-cal margarine	-3 fastfood cheesebgr	-8 beef buiollon	
-2 fast food egg sand	-3 fastfood fried chckn		
-2 chocolate pudding	-3 fried shrimp		
-2 cheese spread	-4 commercial liverwurst		
-3 cream, half & half	-4 commercial bacon		
-3 cream, imitation	-6 pork sausage patty		
-3 sour cream	-8 hot dog		
-5 cream	-19 pepperoni		
-5 whipped cream			
-5 margarine			
-10 butter			

FATS/OILS
Plus Foods

SUGAR
Plus Foods
10 blackstrap
   molasses

ALCOHOL
Plus Foods
10 alcohol free beer

2 near beer

Neutral Foods
0 canned gravy
0 canola oil

Neutral Foods

Neutral Foods

Negative Foods
-1 gravy mixes
-1 lo-cal salad dressing
-1 tartar sauce
-2 salad dressing
-4 mayonnaise
-4 most oils
-5 fast food dressing
-7 onion dip
-10 cononut oil

Negative Foods
-2 lo-cal jelly
-4 diet soft drink
-4 soft drink
-9 jelly
-10 honey
-14 corn syrup
-14 maple syrup
-14 raw sugar
-14 brown sugar
-14 chocolate suace
-16 white sugar
-16 chocolate candy
-33 hard candy

Negative Foods
-10 light beer
-13 beer
-23 wine cooler
-27 gin and tonic
-47 champagne
-47 wine
-103 martini
-150 mint julep
-167 rum
-167 vodka
-177 gin

MODIFIED NUTRIPOINT FOOD LIST

BENSON'S RELAXATION RESPONSE

> When you focus for a short time, gently brushing aside any intrusive thoughts, your mind and body suddenly become a five-star resort in which all service personnel make your restoration and health a priority and are especially concerned with alleviating the harmful effects of stress. This great team of stress-busters and body-relaxers emerges when everyday thoughts and worries are put aside.
>
> —Dr. Herbert Benson, *Timeless Healing*

A Relaxation Response is valuable because it gives your body a mini vacation. And you are in control. You can make the vacation happen anytime you want.

What can be done when you get stressed and the stress has no place to go? You really have two choices. One, use the energy made available by being physically active. Or two, counter the stress with an equal but opposite calming response.

The reason the first approach works is that physical activity in the form of *mild* (less than 60% VO2Max) aerobic exercise, like walking, jogging, swimming, biking, and rowing, helps metabolize the stress hormones and use the energy made available by the "fight or flight" response. The diversion provided by physical activity helps to dissipate the anger, fear, or frustration and replace it with a perception of feeling good about yourself. It also increases confidence in your ability to handle these threatening situations in the future. The biochemical changes resulting from the metabolism of stress hormones and the corresponding release of endorphins contribute to these feelings.

The second method, which works even faster, is to stimulate your Relaxation Response by breathing deeply and calmly. By taking this simple action, you reassert control over your own body.

The well-known author Dr. Herbert Benson took this second method of countering stress to the next level by studying meditation procedures around the world. He found several techniques and principles that have a positive effect on the ability to relax and that result in long-term health benefits by helping to counteract stress. Called the Relaxation Response, Dr. Benson's system provokes a reaction in your body that in every way is opposite from the "fight or flight" response:

- Breathing rate decreases.
- Heart rate decreases.
- Blood pressure decreases.
- Metabolism decreases.
- Oxygen consumption decreases.
- Muscle tension decreases.
- Brain wave frequency decreases.

You don't have to be a yogi or a guru to incorporate the Relaxation Response into your life. Simply follow Dr. Benson's procedure:

1: Chose a focus word, phrase, or sound that makes you feel good (like *beautiful),* one that is firmly rooted in your belief system (like *love),* or one that lets you be passive (like *mmm* or *one).*

To shift the mind from logical, externally oriented

thought, there should be a constant stimulus: a sound, word, or phrase repeated silently or aloud or concentration on breathing. One of the major difficulties in the elicitation of the Relaxation Response is "mind-wandering." This mental device is a way to help break the train of distracting thoughts. You may also focus on slowly tightening and then relaxing muscle groups from your feet to your face.

2: Find a quiet environment, and assume a comfortable position.

You are creating an island of peace and tranquility for yourself. Ideally, you should choose an environment with as few distractions as possible. A quiet room is suitable. The quiet environment makes it easier to eliminate distracting thoughts. Choose a position that you can remain in for at least 10 minutes. Usually a sitting position is recommended because it keeps you from falling asleep. The desired state of consciousness is not sleep, but the same four elements will lead to sleep if you are lying down.

3: Close your eyes, relax, and assume a passive attitude.

Thoughts will come into your head, but let them out again. Don't hold on to them. Distracting thoughts will occur. Don't worry about them. When they occur, disregard them and refocus your attention on your word or phrase or your breathing. Don't worry about how well you are performing the technique, because this may prevent the Relaxation Response from occurring. Adopt a "let it happen" attitude. The passive attitude is perhaps the most important element in eliciting the Relaxation Response.

4: Breathe slowly, and as you exhale, repeat the word, phrase, or sound you have chosen as a focus.

Breathe through your nose. Become aware of your breathing. Breathe easily and naturally. When you inhale, your diaphragm should go down, making your abdomen go out. When you exhale, your diaphragm should go up and your abdomen in. Everyday thoughts may intrude, but let them go and don't judge yourself. Think "whatever," and return to your focus word.

5: Try to do this for about 10 minutes each day, or whenever you feel the need.

If you can't do it for that long, don't worry. Try each day to make it a little part of your day, and you will find yourself making it a part of your day more frequently. Don't worry about the time being exact either. If you can't conveniently time it, just do what you can.

It's better not to practice the Relaxation Response within 2 hours after any meal, since the digestive process seems to interfere with the Relaxation Response.

6: When you are finished, don't get up right away. Let yourself come out of the Relaxation Response gently.

Even if you don't choose to incorporate the Relaxation Response into your daily life, you can still try to take a few deep breaths when you feel harassed. Your body will get the message and start to back off. By changing the mind, you can change the body.

WATER: A GOOD PLACE TO EXERCISE, INJURED OR NOT!

*B*esides being an environment you can come away from feeling relaxed and where you can often have a lot of fun, water is a good place to choose for physical activities for other reasons. Exercising in water allows you to condition your oxygen delivery and consumption system while at the same time allowing:

1. Injuries to heal
2. Weight-bearing joints to recover
3. Muscles to strengthen and tone

Water can be used as a supplement to land training even when you're not injured. You don't lose any conditioning, and you probably gain some strength in the legs and arms. Many people who've worked out in the water say they get better leg-lift and their arms seem easier to move when they return to land. I suggest that you get in the water at least once a week or at least every 2 weeks.

The reason you get these benefits is that working in the water eliminates gravity and presents a resistance. Water is denser than air, and that creates buoyancy. Water has weight, viscosity, and drag, and that creates the resistance.

You can swim, play games, or run in deep water. Again, you are limited only by your imagination. If you work out in deep water, it helps to wear a flotation device. I must admit to a bias in regard to buoyancy belts. When I started a rehabilitation center with Dr. Bruce Becker in Eugene, I wasn't happy with the flotation vests on the market, even the ones intended for the type of training done at our center. They constricted breathing, were irritating, and offered more flotation than needed. So Diahanne Bedortha and I devised the AquaJogger. It costs less than similar products, doesn't interfere with breathing, is light, doesn't cover as much of the body surface, and causes no irritation.

The Aqua Jogger provides you with just enough buoyancy to allow you to concentrate on the motions of training, bicycling, running, or cross-country skiing instead of just trying to keep yourself afloat.

If you are injured, the advantage of running in deep water as opposed to the pool bottom is that you can benefit from the training without aggravating the injury and you can train at a much faster pace. The time and place for training on the pool bottom is when you are ready for the transition from water to land.

There are other advantages to training vertically in deep water. The hydrostatic pressure of the water pushes equally on all surfaces of the body and acts as an auxiliary heart pump. This pressure also acts as a light massage on your body. It's one of the reasons you feel relaxed when you get out of the water. In addition, the temperature of the water will often reduce heat buildup, allowing your body to concentrate on getting blood to the muscles instead of to the skin for cooling. All this results in a lower heart rate at the same apparent effort when working below 75% VO_2Max. Below that intensity you can usually add 10% to your in-water heart rate to get an idea what the on-land heart rate would be. For example, a heart rate of 120 in water is the equivalent of 132 on land. When you work above that intensity, you may find your heart rate increasing more rapidly than usual because as speed of limb movement increases, the drag and resistance increase exponentially. If you move your legs twice as fast, the resistance becomes four times as great.

The techniques of working in the deep water aren't difficult to learn. We start with two tips:

1. Keep an upright posture. If you lean forward you will not get as much benefit from the water as you could. Try to keep the head, neck, buttocks, and legs vertically aligned.
2. Use as much of the water surface as possible. When moving the arms through the water, the palms should always be leading (open and facing ahead when pushing forward, and open and facing backward when pulling backward).

The three primary exercises I recommend are described in the table.

Table 25.1

Exercise	Arms	Legs
Bicycle	As if you were running	As if you were riding a bike
Cross-Country Ski	Straight with relaxed elbow	Straight with relaxed knees
Running	Straight with relaxed elbow or as in breast stroke	As if you were running

Three Primary Exercises

Just as on land, there are an infinite combination of workouts you can do. When someone asks me what to do, I tell them to do exactly what they were going to do on land. I've had distance runners do simulated interval workouts, tempo workouts, and long runs. Sprinters, hurdlers, jumpers, and throwers have worked on starts, hurdle technique, take-offs, and release points. Football players have worked on windsprints and even throwing. Basketball players have put a game on the VCR and pretended they were in it. They would chose a team and do offensive moves when their team was on offense and defensive moves when the team was on defense. Ask yourself, "What would I have planned for land training?" and then do it. You're limited only by your imagination.

How long should the workout be? The same as on land. We have had athletes work for 30 minutes to 2 hours, depending on their workout schedule for any particular day. As a rule, we find that 45 minutes is a minimum effective time because it allows for a warm-up and warm-down period as well as a 30-minute workout.

If you have an injury, you can make it worse in the water. Here are four hints that will help you prevent that from happening:

1. When in doubt, be conservative.
2. If you are injured, stay behind the point of pain. For example, if at 70 degrees of limb movement you have pain, but at 65 you have no pain, only move to 65 degrees.
3. "Nudge" each day. If 65 degrees was comfortable last time, move up a few degrees.
4. When you start feeling good, don't do something foolish or radical. Be satisfied with slow, consistent progression. It is possible to aggravate problems even in water because you're working against resistance.

))))   APPENDIX I   ))))

COMPETITIVE ENDURANCE ATHLETES

The L.E.A.P. program really made a difference for me, even being a varsity wrestler. I can monitor my optimal amount of energy use and maintain those limits.
—Jeremy Ensrud, University of Oregon wrestler, ranked #2 in US

L.E.A.P. is beneficial for people at any training or competitive level. To balance challenge and recovery it is important to be able to estimate the amount of energy it is most efficient for you to convert each week and the actual amount you are converting in your workouts. L.E.A.P. will help you keep your energy conversion and recovery balanced. If you are training at a high level and for eventual competition, L.E.A.P. can help you get to your competitions in the best possible condition.

There are two ways L.E.A.P. can help in addition to the information in the book. First, there are some coefficients you can use with your ECPs formula that will give you more credit for energy converted during some special workouts like fartlek, tempo, and intervals, and for races (defined below).

Second, in this appendix I provide some general guidelines I share with the athletes I coach. These guidelines are applicable to any endurance activity. They have been used successfully with runners, swimmers, cross-country skiers, and a jet boat driver who won the world amateur championship in that sport.

When I speak about training, in addition to the actual workouts and methods of working out I also mean:

- Diet

Your diet can help you recover and therefore train better, which will improve performance. There is no diet that will magically enhance your performance. In Appendix F I discussed the diet I encourage the athletes I work with to eat. It is balanced, provides enough nutrient-rich foods, is not restrictive, and can be very enjoyable. There are many special diets that are promoted, and I am sure some are more specific than what I suggest. But in the crowded diet marketplace, it's too easy to get a bad one that is promoted heavily. It takes significant experience and time to research claims to insure that a special diet will be beneficial. Therefore, until I am better educated about special diets, I will stick to what I know will help promote recovery, promote adaptation, and do no harm.

If you are making sure you are getting a balanced diet and are still hungry, it's OK to eat high-calorie snacks like some ice cream or chocolate chip cookies.

- Dietary Supplements

As with diets, there are many different supplements and even more claims that supplements will improve your performance. I have a big box of unopened advertisements for dietary supplements. I'm sure some will aid performance. I'm sure some will take your money and give you nothing back. I wish I had time to investigate the claims and understand the mechanisms by which the supplements work. But I don't have that kind of time.

So I say to athletes that if a supplement company claims to have scientific proof but does not cite the literature from which they determined this proof, dismiss the claim.

I also tell them to look at labels. Recently a company wanted an athlete I coach to endorse their total nutrient recovery supplement. A look at the label showed no protein in the supplement. It can't be a full recovery drink without protein.

Finally, I tell them to know the supplement dealer or brand. Too often dealers or brands just want to make money and use shortcuts like fillers, adulterated ingredients, and mislabeling.

I divide supplements into three categories: dietary supplements, recovery drinks, and performance enhancers. Those I have found useful are listed in the table below. I do not work for any of the companies mentioned, do not get any commissions, and they don't even know I am making these suggestions. I mention them only because I have found them useful and suggest that my athletes use them. There are other supplements that I am sure are useful but have only limited experience with them.

Table 26.1

DIETARY	Suggestions	Value	Contact
Vitamin C	a.m./p.m. 1-5 g	Illness, injury, adrenaline	
Multivitamin	As directed	Nutrient insurance	
Vitamin E	As directed	Antioxidant	
Liver (organic; desiccated /extract)	As directed	Red blood cells	
Echinacea	Not constantly, as directed	Immune enhancer	
RECOVERY DRINK			
Exceleration	As directed within 30 minutes after workout	Total nutrients	Excel Sports Science, Eugene, OR
PERFORMANCE AID			
Boston Sports Supplement	1 packet 30 minutes before hard effort	Helps nerve transmission by preventing fall in plasma choline	InterNutria, Framingham, MA
Access Bar	1 bar 30 minutes before hard effort	Balanced energy release	Melaleuca, Idaho Falls, ID
Creatine	As directed	ATP recycling	Experimental and Applied Sciences, Golden, CO
Caffeine	< 200 mg 20 minutes before hard effort	Central nervous system stimulant	

Dietary Supplements

- Sleep/Relaxation

See Sleep in Chapter 5 and Appendix G on the Relaxation Response.

- Massage

Massage is one of the best investments you can make. It

will speed recovery by promoting blood flow, prevent small stress points from becoming major problems, and enhance proper postural and biomechanical alignment. A massage at least once every 2 weeks potentiates your ability to recover and prevent injuries. When you are injured, it can help your body heal faster.

- Warm-Up and Warm-Down

Warm-up reduces muscle and connective tissue viscosity, reducing the risk of injury. Warm-down helps remove the products of activity and speeds your recovery process.

- Flexibility

Nonballistic stretching, which is a static stretch without bouncing movements, before a workout helps lengthen the muscle fibers. Lengthened fibers help prevent injuries to muscles, ligaments, and tendons and improve biomechanical efficiency. The same type of stretching after a workout further serves to lengthen the muscle fibers and promote recovery

- Weight/Strength Training

Developing balanced strength in your body will help prevent injuries and enhance your performance. When you select a strength training program, you should first emphasize balance of muscle groups, and only then should you add some exercises for your speciality.

Strength training should be done after your harder workouts in the week for two reasons. First, your cardiovascular system is already functioning at a higher level, and by lifting now you will keep it at a high level and gain cardiovascular benefits as you lift. Second, easy days should be easy. If you lift on your easy days, they will not be easy and will impede long-term adaptation.

- Technique

Working on technique improves your efficiency. Improved efficiency allows you to move faster using less energy. You can practice technique during easy, steady, fartlek, and long runs.

During races, good athletes associate with their feelings rather than dissociate from them. They are thinking about the task at hand and evaluating their feelings, pace, and technique, as opposed to trying to keep their minds on factors not associated with the race. Improving technique in training helps you associate better in races by focusing on efficient biomechanics.

- Illness Prevention

You can improve your ability to prevent illness if you:
1. Dress appropriately. Be too warm rather than too cold. You can always take clothes off.
2. Warm up properly and go through the workout without lag time.
3. Stay within workout parameters.
4. Hydrate during a workout, if needed, and within 30 minutes after completion with a protein/carbohydrate recovery drink.
5. Keep warm between the end of your workout and your shower.
6. Get a warm shower as soon as possible after your workout.
7. Follow a good diet, including plenty of water.
8. Get to bed about the same time each night, and get the amount of sleep you need.

There are four simple indicators that can tell you if you have recovered from your most recent physical or emotional challenges, and they can be determined within minutes of awakening. You can use them in a very orderly way, or you can just be aware of them. They can help you stay healthy.

Table 26.2

Recovery Indicator	Not Fully Recovered If...
A.M. Heart Rate	> 110% of Normal
A.M. Body Weight	< 97% of Normal
Time to Bed	> 40 Minutes Later Than Normal
Perceived Hours Slept	< 90% of Normal

If one indicator is abnormal, monitor yourself during the workout and be prepared to back off. If two are abnormal, plan an easier day. If three or more are abnormal, take the day off or do any physical activity at very low intensity.

- Keep a Diary

WORKOUT PHILOSOPHIES AND PROGRAM OUTLINES

It is my feeling that you can race up to almost 90% or 95% of your potential with maximum steady state training only. Maximum steady state training is safe training. You can recover from this type of training within 24 hours. It is training that enhances your ability to deliver and consume oxygen so that you do not significantly engage anaerobic metabolism.

Maximum steady state training is training between 80% and 85% VO2Max as often as your body allows. You can go as low as 70% VO2Max and still get beneficial results.

Described below are three general programs:

1. 13 weeks to peak
2. 26 weeks to peak
3. 39 weeks to peak

The general philosophy is that you pick one race where you would like to do your best. Call it The Race. All training is directed toward that race. You can race any other time you want as long as you do not allow yourself to get too emotionally involved. All other races should be run in a manner that challenges but does not overwhelm you; that is, a tempo pace. Tempo pace is a pace where you definitely feel challenged, but you are still in control of your body. It is not in control of you. When you finish these tempo efforts, you should be tired *but* exhilarated, not tired *and* exhausted. In the 13-weeks-to-peak program, you can have one other race where you push harder than tempo pace. In the 26-week program, you can have two other races where you push yourself harder than tempo pace. In the 39-week program, you can have four or five races where you push yourself harder than tempo pace.

Table 26.3 outlines the emphasis of the training during the weeks leading up to The Race.

Table 26.3

13-Weeks	26 Weeks	39 Weeks	Training Emphasis	Primary Training Goal
Weeks 1-8	Weeks 1-18	Weeks 1-30	Steady State	Raise Aerobic Base
Week 9	Weeks 19-20	Weeks 29-31	Hill Sessions[1]	Leg Strength
Week 10	Weeks 21-22	Weeks 32-34	Long Intervals[2]	Stimulate Anaerobic Enzymes
Week 11	Weeks 23-24	Weeks 35-37	Short Intervals[3]	Race Sharpening
Week 12	Week 25	Week 38	Some Speed and Rest	Peak for Race[4]
Week 13	Week 26	Week 39	Active Rest	Recovery

Training Emphasis

[1] Find a hill that is fairly flat at top and bottom. The incline should be more than gradual but less than steep. If it is grass or dirt, so much the better.

Table 26.4 shows you what percentage of your ECPs you should try to attain on a 5-, 6-, and 7-day workout week.

Table 26.4

Days/ Week Active	Day 1	Day 2	Day 3	Day 4	Day 5	Day 6	Day 7
5	26	12	20		22		20
6	24	12	16		20	12	16
7	22	10	15	10	18	10	15

Percentage of ECPs per Day

After you warm up, run up a 100-meter hill four times, increasing your pace just a little each time. At the top, jog for 3 minutes, and then stride down the hill at a smooth, controlled pace. At the bottom of the hill, do four 50-meter strides. Swimmers won't have hills, but the idea is to try to make the effort against gravity or some other force. Cyclists may want to increase the distances for the hills accordingly. These are general guidelines. You may want to do less or more or progress a little each time you try them. If you are doing a 39-week-to-peak program, you may want to find a longer hill for the last week. Just remember, if in doubt, be conservative!

2 Long intervals should be between 400 meters and 1000 meters or their time/distance equivalents on bikes, skis, or water. The total distance for a workout should be between 1.5 and 2 times race distance but never longer than 5000 meters. The pace should be no faster than your projected race pace. The exception in pace and distance is a workout where you run three to five times 5 minutes at your 5000-meter pace. You should be nearly or fully recovered before you start your next interval segment. A good way to determine paces is to get *Oxygen Power: Performance Tables for Distance Runners,* by Dr. Jack Daniels, 948 Walden Pond Lane, Cortland, N.Y. 13045. I have used his tables extensively.

3 Short intervals should be between 100 and 300 meters or their time/distance equivalents on bikes, skis, or water. The total distance should be no longer than 1800 meters. The pace can start at a little slower than race pace and gradually become faster with each succeeding interval. At least half of the intervals should be run faster than race pace. Starting your first interval at a slower pace and running your last interval at the fastest pace is called cutting down, or cutdowns.

4 During the peak week it is very important to make sure you do not overdo. I have seen many good races come after rest. I have seen few come after overwork. The saying "When in doubt, be conservative!" is an important training concept and especially applies during the peak week.

The following table shows the type of workout to do on a given day.

Two comments apply to all periods or all workouts. First, if you want to do a second workout in a day, it should be considered a recovery workout. The duration of a recovery workout should be between 10 and 20 minutes. The intensity of a recovery workout should be no more than 60% VO_2Max.

Second, anytime you want to use deep water for a recovery workout or to cross-train instead of your planned workout, never hesitate. Working out in the water is very beneficial. You will gain cardiovascular fitness while at the same time your muscles, joints, and bones will be healing.

Table 26.5

Period	Day 1	Day 2	Day 3	Day 4	Day 5	Day 6	Day 7
Steady State	Steady State	Steady State w/6x10 sec Technique	Steady State	Steady State	Steady State	Steady State	Steady State w/5 minutes Fartlek[5] or Tempo Effort
Hills	Steady State	Steady State	Hills	Steady State	Hills	Steady State	Steady State w/5 minutes Fartlek on Hills or Tempo[6] effort
Long Intervals	Steady State	Steady State	Long Intervals	Steady State	Long Intervals	Steady State	Steady State w/5 minutes Fartlek or Controlled Race Effort
Short Intervals	Easy Steady State	Steady State	Short Intervals	Steady State	Short Intervals	Steady State	Tempo or Controlled Race Effort
Peak	Very Easy Steady State	3-4x300	Jog	3-4x150	Jog	Jog	The Race[7]

Percentage of ECPs per Day

---

5 Literally speedplay. In this workout you play at varying the pace. There is no set time to do a faster pace. You might decide, I think I'll run a little faster between the next two telephone poles. In the steady state period on your Day 7 workout, for example, you would inject segments that total 5 minutes of faster pace in the total workout.

6 You are challenged but very much in control of your effort and you should be able to finish the effort at the same pace you started it. However, if you would go just a little faster, lactate production would exceed lactate removal, which decreases pH, and your body would become increasingly more in control as it tried to maintain homeostasis.

7 This is the race you have been training for. Now the saying changes in one small but important way. "When in doubt, be conservative, unless you are in doubt about what to do during the last 35% of The Race; then be aggressive." In racing, start challenged but controlled. But with about 20% of the race to go, make sure you push yourself.

SPECIAL L.E.A.P. COEFFICIENTS
FOR SERIOUS ATHLETES

The table below provides some additional coefficients for serious athletes. Tempo efforts, fartlek, intervals, and races have an emotional component that demands the mobilization of additional resources and energy conversion. The coefficients in the following table give you energy conversion credit for these additional challenges to your body. Multiply your ECPs by these coefficients to get revised ECPs for these types of workouts.

For example, if you did a moderate tempo effort and earned 60 ECPs, you would multiply 60 by 1.18 to get your revised ECPs of 71.

Table 26.6

Fartlek /Tempo Race	Easy Effort	Moderate Effort	Hard Effort
Fartlek Coef	1.02	1.07	1.15
Tempo Coef	1.13	1.18	1.27
Race Coef	2.30	2.41	2.59

Interval	>90% VO2Max	>95% VO2Max	100% VO2Max
Interval Coef	1.71	1.80	1.93
Interval Recovery	**Full**	**Moderate**	**Short**
Recovery Coef	.75	.85	.95

Time Continuous Workout	> 40 min	40-60 min	> 60 min
Time Coef	1.00	1.02	1.05

Coefficients for Serious Athletes

STRENGTH TRAINING

Strength training is an important aspect of fitness. While this type of training is usually associated with a higher level of athletics, it has been shown that by maintaining strength as we age our health is significantly enhanced. Even elderly citizens who have not worked out for years, have experienced improvements in the muscular and skeletal systems when engaging in a strength training program. These improvements resulted in a more independent lifestyle.

Following is a basic strength program that emphasizes major muscle groups. Anyone can benefit from these exercises and, by paying attention to starting weights and/or repetitions, can proceed in a safe manner. There are many ways to approach strength training and if you develop an interest in progressing to more complex programs you would be wise to seek guidance at a respected health club or from a well-educated professional. A specialist in strength training and movement, especially for mature and senior citizens, is Dr. Laura VanHarn at the Phytness Connection, 6116 LaSalle Ave., Oakland, CA 94611. Phone 510-339-6546. Email laura@phytness.com.

Each of the 12 exercises below are easily done at any health club. By doing the movements with no (0) weight, and/or supplementing some exercises with light dumbbells, all the exercises can be done at home.

Safety first! When in doubt be conservative. Use less weight rather than more. Do fewer repetitions rather than more. If using weights, lift every other day, not every day. Progress slowly.

Table 27.1

6 Major Areas	Movement	Description	Sample Exercise	Equipment	Starting Weight	Repetitions
Arms Chest Upper Back	Arms Overhead	Arms push weight from shoulders	Military Press	Barbell	0 to 1/4 body weight	8 10 12
	Arms Back Down	Arms pull weight from overhead	Pulldowns	Pulldown Machine (chin bar)	0 to full body weight	8 to 12
Arms Chest Upper Back	Arms Outfront	Arms push weight out front	Pushups or Knee Pushups	None	0 to full body weight	8 to 12
	Arms Back In	Arms pull weight back in	Rowing	Pulldown Machine w/Rowing attached	0 to 1/2 body weight	8 to 12
Abdomen Lower back	Trunk Bent Forward	Move trunk closer to knees	Situps (Crunch)	None	0	12 to 20
	Trunk Straight	Move trunk away from knees	Sitback	Weight Plate (hold plate to chest, bend and straighten	0 to 25 pd	12 to 20
Buttocks Groin	Legs Straight	Legs push weight away from body	Leg Press	None or Leg Press Machine	0 to full body weight	12 to 20
	Legs Bent	Legs raised toward body	Bent Leg Raises	None or Roman Chair	0	12 to 20
Thigh Hamstrings	Knee Straight	Knees from bent to straight	Quadricep Extension	None (lie on back, bend/straighten 1 leg at a time	0	8 to 12
	Knee Bent	Knees from straight to bent	Hamstring Curl	Hamstring Curl	0 to 1/4 body weight	8 to 12
Lower Legs Ankles	Ankle Extended	Push toes away from body	Toe Raises	None or leg Press Machine	0 to full body weight	12 to 20
	Ankle Flexed	Pull toes towards body	Isometric Ankle Flex	None (pull toes towards knees hold 10 sec)	0	3 to 5

FLEXIBILTY

*F*lexibility is also an important aspect of fitness. As with strength, flexibility programs can be much more involved than the sample I provide. If you want more information, a good source is a book, *Active Isolated Stretching*, by Jim and Phil Wharton. To order the book call 1-800-240-9805.

Below are five easy stretches that address major areas of the body. GENTLY hold each position for a slow 10-count or a moderate 25 count. You can do each once or repeat as often as feels comfortable.

Table 28.1

5 Basic Stretches	Description

4 Position Neck	The positions are
	   look up
	   look down
	   look left
	   look right

Trunk Twist & Bend	Right arm straight up past your ear
	   left arm straight down past your hip,
	   bend and gently twist left.
	   Reverse arm positions and stretch right

Back of Body	With legs shoulder width and slightly bent, gently bend over and drop hands toward floor
Front of Body	With legs shoulder width, stretch both arms overhead and gently lean back.

Achilles and Calves	Face a wall. Legs shoulder width, heels on floor.
	   With arms straight, put hands on wall. Lean
	   toward wall by bending arms.

AMA SPECIAL COMMUNICATION

Several years ago a Special Communication appeared in the *Journal of the American Medical Association*. When I read it the L.E.A.P. concept was already 8 years old, and it seemed to me that the L.E.A.P. philosophy coincided with the observations and suggestions put forth in the article. The article excerpts are in plain print and L.E.A.P.'s philosophy, as recorded in 1987, is in bold print.

February 1, 1995. Special communication–physical activity and public health. *Journal of the American Medical Association* 273(5):402–7.

Millions of Americans remain essentially sedentary. If Americans who lead sedentary lives would adopt a more active lifestyle, there would be an enormous benefit to the public's health and well-being.

L.E.A.P.'s original, and still the most important, target is the 45 million people who believe in the benefits of activity, but are not yet consistently active.

The current low-participation rate may be due in part to the misconception of many people that to reap health benefits they must engage in vigorous, continuous exercise. The scientific evidence clearly demonstrates that regular moderate-intensity physical activity provides substantial health benefits.

The L.E.A.P. program has emphasized the benefits of regular, moderate-intensity physical activity.

It now appears that the majority of these health benefits can be gained by performing moderate-intensity physical activities outside of formal exercise programs. . . . Physical activity is any bodily movement produced by skeletal muscles that results in energy expenditure.

L.E.A.P. said, "Activity encompasses all physical endeavors, not just exercise. An active lifestyle can include exercise, but is not limited to it."

L.E.A.P. has encouraged the use of the words "activity" instead of "exercise," and encouraged people to participate in physical activity they enjoy. With L.E.A.P. over 150 activities can be used to contribute to the health benefits of physical activity.

Accumulation of physical activity in intermittent, short bouts is considered an appropriate approach to achieving the activity goal. Health benefits of physical activity are linked principally to total amount of physical activity performed.

The L.E.A.P. program encourages recording any physical activity that has converted energy in the L.E.A.P. Log.

Every U.S. adult should accumulate 30 minutes or more of moderate-intensity physical activity on most, preferably all, days of the week.

L.E.A.P. sets Risk Reduction, Success Zone, and Optimal ECPs goals. The Success Zone goals always fall within the "30 minutes of moderate-intensity activity most days of the week" guideline.

The 30 minutes of activity should be accumulated during the course of the day. Intermittent activity also confers substantial benefits. Therefore the recommended 30 minutes can be accumulated in short bouts of activity.

L.E.A.P. accounts for all physical activities and for any duration.

Those who do not engage in regular physical activity should begin by incorporating a few minutes of increased activity into their day, building gradually to 30 minutes per day of activity.

L.E.A.P. has the Safe Minimum and Risk Reduction goals and establishes your Week 1 Optimal ECPs based on your physical characteristics, lifestyle, and current activity pattern. It then provides a method for you to progress at your pace.

A lack of time is the most commonly cited barrier to participation in physical activity, and injury is a common reason for stopping regular activity.

L.E.A.P. considers time availability in the autobiography and uses this in constructing an Optimal Goal. This goal, based upon many factors, is structured in a way that helps prevent injury due to early overexuberance.

Confidence in the ability to be physically active and enjoyment of activity are strongly related to participation.

L.E.A.P. helps you set goals which you can be confident are the right goals for you. L.E.A.P. encourages participation in a wide range of enjoyable activities.

Low-to-moderate intensity physical activities are more likely to be continued than high-intensity activities.

L.E.A.P. encourages you to be physically active at a level you can handle and enjoy. L.E.A.P. even encourages serious athletes to stay below anaerobic training levels on most occasions. Your goals can be attained with the intensity that is most comfortable for you.

Family and friends can be role models, provide encouragement, or be companions during physical activity.

L.E.A.P. considers the support of family and friends in setting goals, and encourages you to cultivate their support.

Self-regulatory skills, such as goal setting, self-monitoring of progress, and self-reinforcement, contribute to continued physical activity.

L.E.A.P. enhances the person's ability to regulate their own program by allowing them to participate in the goal-setting process, by enabling them to monitor themselves, and by reinforcing their activity via quick, accurate feedback.

There is a clear association between total daily or weekly caloric expenditure and cardiovascular disease mortality.

L.E.A.P. enables the user to see how many calories they converted every time they were active and encourages the person to eventually reach Paffenbarger's caloric conversion numbers of at least 500 to 3000 calories per week via physical activity.

Physicians and other health professionals should routinely counsel patients to adopt and maintain regular physical activity. Patients respect physicians' advice and change their exercise behavior as a result. Inadequate reimbursement, limited physician knowledge of the benefits of physical activity, lack of training in physical activity counseling, and inadequate knowledge of effective referral are barriers to achieving these goals.

L.E.A.P. can make any doctor or other health professional a fitness expert. Insurance reimbursements for this preventive service would save billions of dollars.

Health professionals should be physically active not only to benefit their own health, but to make more creditable their endorsement of an active lifestyle.

L.E.A.P. can make it easy for health professionals, even on their busy schedules, to improve their activity habits.

WHAT IS A WORKOUT?
BY GEORGE ALLEN

A workout is 25 percent perspiration and 75 percent determination. Stated another way, it is one part physical exertion and three parts self-discipline. Doing it is easy once you get started.

A workout makes you better today than you were yesterday. It strengthens the body, relaxes the mind, and toughens the spirit. When you work out regularly, your problems diminish and your confidence grows.

A workout is a personal triumph over laziness and procrastination. It is a badge of a winner—the mark of an organized, goal-oriented person who has taken charge of his, or her, destiny.

A workout is a wise use of time and an investment in excellence. It is a way of preparing for life's challenges and proving to yourself that you have what it takes to do what is necessary.

A workout is a key that helps unlock the door of opportunity and success. Hidden within each of us is an extraordinary force. Physical and mental fitness are the triggers that can release it.

A workout is a form of rebirth. When you finish a good workout, you don't simply feel better. You feel better about yourself.

George Allen was a very successful football coach of the Los Angeles Rams and Washington Redskins. He believed firmly in the benefits of an active lifestyle and lived his life as an example.

L.E.A.P. COMPUTER PROGRAM/DIARY

*T*here is an easy-to-use computer version of the L.E.A.P. program that will also do all the evaluations and calculations for you and your family.

To find out more about the L.E.A.P. Computer Program or Diary, call:

1-800-SAY-L.E.A.P.
(1-800-729-5327)

or contact LEAP on the internet at:

www.LeapInc.com

WEEK 1 COEFFICENT EXAMPLE

W1Coef saves you a lot of work by eliminating many terms you need to cancel out. If you want to see how it was computed you can follow the example of Marlene.

Components of Formula:
1. Recommended days per week of activity based upon Activity Category.
   For Marlene, frequency = 5 days/week

2. Recommended minutes per day of activity based upon Activity Category.
   For Marlene, duration = 50 minutes/day

3. Recommended average intensity of activity based upon Activity Category.
   For Marlene, average %VO2Max =74%, which = ICoef of 1.175

4. Perfect Support/Time Score
   A perfect Support/Time Score = 3.25

5. A number which converts milliliters to liters, pounds to kilograms, and which is modified to account for the exponential nature of various intensities, durations, and VO2Max's.

1000 ml/liter x 2.2pounds/kg x .88 = 1936 ml-pounds/liter-kg

The formula looks like this:

(5 days/wk x 50 min/day x 1.175) ÷ (1936 ml lb/liter kg x 3.25) =

.047 min liters kg/wk ml lb = Marlene's Week 1 Coefficient

When her Week 1 Optimal ECPs are computed it looks like this:

VO2Max Coefficient x Support/Time Number x Weight x Week 1 Coefficient

21.41ml/kg/min x 2.25 x 143 lb x .047 min liters kg/wk ml lb = 324 liter/week = 324 ECPs

Andrew, G.M., et al. 1981. Reasons for dropout from exercise programs in post-coronary patients. *Medicine and Science in Sports and Exercise* 13:164–68.

Andrews, J.G. 1983. Biochemical measures of muscular effort. *Medicine and Science in Sports and Exercise* 15: 199–207.

Appenzeller, O., and R. Atkinson, eds. 1977. *Medicine and sport.* Vol. 12 of *Health aspects of endurance training.* Basel: S. Karger.

———. 1981. *Sports medicine: fitness, training, injuries.* Munich: Urban & Schwarzenberg.

Argov, Z., et al. 1988. Detection of muscle injury in humans with ^{31}P magnetic resonance spectroscopy. *Muscle and Nerve* 2: 212–216.

Asmussen, E. 1979. Muscle fatigue. *Medicine and Science in Sports* 11:313–21.

Astrand, P.O., and K. Rodahl. 1977. *Textbook of work physiology.* New York: McGraw-Hill.

Baack, Lawrence J., ed. 1975. *The worlds of Brutus Hamilton.* Los Altos, Calif.: Tafnews Press.

Badenhop, D.T., et al. 1983. Physiological adjustments to higher- or lower-intensity exercise in elders. *Medicine and Science in Sports and Exercise* 15:496–502.

Bailey, C. 1977. Fit or fat . Boston: Houghton Mifflin Company.

———. 1994. Smart Exercise . Boston: Houghton Mifflin Company.

Bannister, E.W., and S.R. Brown. 1968. The relative energy requirements of physical activity. In *Exercise physiology*, edited by H.B. Falls. New York: Academic Press.

Barnes, L. 1980. Measuring anaerobic threshold simplified. *Physician and Sportsmedicine* 8(7):15–16.

Barnes-Svarney, P., ed. 1995. *The New York Public Library science desk reference.* New York: MacMillan.

Bechtel, S. 1993. The Practical encyclopedia of sex and health. Emmaus, PA.: Rodale Press.

Benson, H. 1975. *The relaxation response*. New York: William Morrow.

———. 1984. *Beyond the relaxation response*. New York: Times Books.

———. 1989. *The mind/body effect*. New York: Avon Books.

———. 1994. *Timeless healing*. New York: Scribners.

Berg, A., and G. Haralambie. 1978. Changes in serum creatine kinase and hexose phosphate isomerase activity with exercise duration. *European Journal of Applied Physiology* 39:191–201.

Birk, T.J., and C.A. Birk. 1987. Use of ratings of perceived exertion for exercise prescription. *Sports Medicine* 4:1–8.

Blanksby, B.A., and P.W. Reidy. 1988. Heart rate and estimated energy expenditure during ballroom dancing. *British Journal of Sports Medicine* 22:57–60.

Bompa, T.O. 1983. *Theory and methodology of training*. Dubuque, Iowa: Kendall/Hunt Publishers.

Booth, F. W., and P.D. Gollnick. 1983. Effects of disuse on the structure and function of skeletal muscle. *Medicine and Science in Sports and Exercise* 15:415–20.

Borg, G. 1970. Perceived exertion as an indicator of somatic stress. *Scandnavian Journal of Rehabilitation Medicine* 2:92–98.

———. 1982. Psychophysical bases of perceived exertion. *Medicine and Science in Sports and Exercise* 14:377–81.

———. 1985. *An introduction to Borg's RPE scale*. Ithaca, N.Y.: Movement Publications.

Borg, G., P. Hassmen, and M. Lagerstrom. 1987. Perceived exertion related to heart rate and blood lactate during arm and leg exercise. *European Journal of Applied Physiology* 65:679–85.

Borg, G., G. Ljunggren, and R. Ceci. 1985. The increase of perceived exertion on aches and pains in the legs, heart rate and blood lactate during exercise on a bicycle ergometer. *European Journal of Applied Physiology* 54:343–49.

Borysewicz, E. 1985. *Bicycle road racing: Complete program for training and competition*. Brattleboro, Vt.: Vitesse Press.

Bouchard, C., et al. 1979. Specificity of maximal aerobic power. *European Journal of Applied Physiology* 40:85–93.

Bouchard, C., et al. 1990. *Exercise, fitness and health*. Champaign, Ill.: Human Kinetics Books.

Bowerman, W.J. 1974. *Coaching track and field*. Boston: Houghton Mifflin.

Bowerman, W.J., and W.E. Harris. 1967. *Jogging, a physical fitness program for all ages*. New York: Grosset & Dunlap.

Bray, G.A. 1983. The energetics of obesity. *Medicine and Science in Sports and Exercise* 15:32–40.

Brooks, C.M. 1987. Adult participation in physical activities requiring moderate to high levels of energy expenditure. *Physician and Sportsmedicine* 15(4):119–32.

Brooks, G.A. 1985. Anaerobic threshold: Review of the concept and directions for future research. *Medicine and Science in Sports and Exercise* 17:22–31.

Brooks, G.A. 1986. The lactate shuttle during exercise and recovery. *Medicine and Science in Sports and Exercise* 18:360–68.

Brooks, G.A., and T.D. Fahey. 1984. *Exercise physiology, human bioenergics and its applications*. New York: John Wiley & Sons.

Brown, R.L. 1984. Running smart. *The Runner*, January.

———. 1984. Das training von Mary Decker. *Leicht Athletik*, April.

———. 1986. Listen to your body talk. *Runner's World*, May.

———. 1992. ^{31}P Metabolic responses to activity of nonspecifically trained muscle tissue in elite endurance athletes and in healthy, sedentary subjects as observed by ^{31}Pmagnetic resonance spectroscopy. Ph.D. diss., University of Oregon.

Brownell, K.D. 1984. Behavioral and psychological aspects of motivation to exercise. *International Journal of Sports Medicine* 5(Suppl):69–70.

Burdon, J.G.W., K.J. Killian, and E.J.M. Campbell. 1982. Effect of ventilatory drive on the perceived magnitude of added loads to breathing. *Journal of Applied Physiology* 53:901–7.

Canadian Armed Forces. 1988. *Express: The exercise prescription*. Toronto: MacMillan of Canada.

Cafarelli, E. 1982. Peripheral contributions to the perception of effort. *Medicine and Science in Sports and Exercise* 14:382–89.

Cantwell, J.D. 1986. Cardiac rehabilitation in the mid–1980's. *Physician and Sportsmedicine* 14(4):89–96.

Carton, R.L., and E.C. Rhodes. 1985. A critical review of the literature on ratings scales for perceived exertion. *Sports Medicine* 2:198–222.

Clarkson, P.M., and I. Tremblay. 1988. Exercise-induced muscle damage, repair, and adaptation in humans. *Journal of Applied Physiology* 65:1–6.

Cohen, F. 1985. Stress and bodily illness. In *Stress and coping–An anthology*, edited by A. Monat and R.S. Lazarus. 2d ed. New York: Columbia University Press.

Conconi, F., et al. 1982. Determination of the anaerobic threshold by a noninvasive field test in runners. *Journal of Applied Physiology* 52:869–73.

Cooper, K.H. 1968. A means of assessing maximal oxygen intake. *JAMA* 203:135–38.

———. 1968. *Aerobics*. New York: Bantam Books.

———. 1970. *The new aerobics*. New York: Bantam Books.

———. 1982. *The aerobics program for total well-being*. New York: Bantam Books.

Costill, D.L. 1979. *A scientific approach to distance running*. Mountain View, Calif.: Track & Field News.

———. 1986. *Inside running: Basics of sports physiology*. Carmel, Ind.: Benchmark Press.

Costill, D.L., and E.L. Fox. 1969. Energetics of marathon running. *Medicine and Science in Sports* 1:81–86.

Costill, D.L., P.J. Cahill, and D. Eddy. 1967. Metabolic responses to sub-maximal exercise in three water temperatures. *Journal of Applied Physiology* 22:628–32.

Cote, R.W., and J.H. Wilmore. 1986. A practical assessment of body composition in young women. *Journal of Sports Medicine* 26:427–30.

Coutts, K.D., and J.L. Stogryn. 1987. Aerobic and anaerobic power of Canadian wheelchair track athletes. *Medicine and Science in Sports and Exercise* 19:62–65.

Cronan, T.L., and E.T. Howley. 1974. The effect of training on epinephrine and norepinephrine excretion. *Medicine and Science in Sports* 6:122–25.

Cureton, T.K. Jr. 1965. Physical fitness and dynamic health. New York: The Dial Press.

Czajkowski, W. A simple method to control fatigue in endurance training. In *Exercise and sport biology*, edited by P.V. Komi. Vol. 12 of *International series on sport sciences*. Champaign, Ill. Human Kinetics.

Daniels, J.T., R.A. Yarbrough, and C. Foster. 1978. Changes in VO_2 max and running performance with training. *European Journal of Applied Physiology* 39:249–54.

Daniels, J.T. 1979. *Oxygen power: performance tables for distance runners*, 948 Walden Pond Lane, Cortland, NY, 13045

deVries, H.A. *Physiology for physical education and athletics*. Dubuque, Iowa: Wm. C. Brown.

diPrampero, P.E. 1986. The energy cost of human locomotion on land and in water. *International Journal of Sports Medicine* 7:55–72.

Dishman, R.K. 1982. Health psychology and exercise adherence. *Quest* 33(2):66–180.

———. 1984. Motivation and exercise adherence. In *Psychological foundations of sport,* edited by J.M. Silva and R.S. Weinberg. Champaign, Ill. Human Kinetics.

———. 1986. Exercise compliance: A new view for public health. *Physician and Sportsmedicine* 14(5):127–42.

———. ed. 1988. *Exercise adherence: Its impact on public health.* Champaign, Ill: Human Kinetics.

Dishman, R.K., and L.R. Gettman. 1980. Psychobiologic influences on exercise adherence. *Journal of Sport Psychology* 2:295–310.

Dishman, R.K., W. Ickes, and W.P. Morgan. 1980. Self-motivation and adherence to habitual physical activity. *Journal of Applied Social Psychology* 10(2):115–32.

Dishman, R.K., J.F. Sallis, and D.R. Orenstein. 1985. The determinants of physical activity and exercise. *Public Health Reports* 100(2):158–71.

Dishman, R.K., et al. 1987. Using perceived exertion to prescribe and monitor exercise training heart rate. *International Journal of Sports Medicine* 8:208–13.

Doherty, J.K. 1964. *Modern training for running.* Englewood Cliffs, N.J.: Prentice Hall.

Dorociak, J.J., and J.K. Nelson. 1983. The 1 mile and 2 mile runs as measures of cardiovascular fitness in college women. *Journal of Sports Medicine* 23:322–25.

Dressendorfer, R.H., C.E. Wade, and J.H. Scaff. 1985. Increased morning heart rate in runners: A valid sign of overtraining? *Physician and Sportsmedicine* 13(8):77–86.

Durant, R.H., E.V. Dover, and B.S. Alpert. 1983. An evaluation of five indices of physical working capacity in children. *Medicine and Science in Sports and Exercise* 15:83–87.

Dustman, R.E., et al. 1984. Aerobic exercise training and improved neuropsychological function of older individuals. *Neurobiology of Aging* 5:35–42.

Dwyer, J., and R. Bybee. 1983. Heart rate indices of the anaerobic threshold. *Medicine and Science in Sports and Exercise* 15:72–76.

Eichner, E.R. 1988. Circadian timekeepers in sports. *Physician and Sportsmedicine* 16(2):79–85.

Epstein, Y., L.A. Stroschein, and K.B. Pandolf. 1987. Predicting metabolic cost of running with and without backpack loads. *European Journal of Applied Physiology* 56:495–500.

Epstein, Y., et al. 1988. External load can alter the energy cost of prolonged exercise. *European Journal of Applied Physiology* 57:243–47.

Evans, T., ed. 1989. *The Stanford health & exercise handbook.* Champaign, Ill: Leisure Press.

Farwell, R.R., and J.L. Mayhew. 1983. Task specificity in the relationship of predicted VO2 max and run performance. *Journal of Sports Medicine* 23:286–90.

Fitts, R.H., et al. 1984. The effect of ageing and exercise on skeletal muscle function. *Mechanisms of Ageing and Development* 27:161–72.

Fohrenbach, R., A. Mader, and W. Hollmann. 1987. Determination of endurance capacity and prediction of exercise intensities for training and competition in marathon runners. *International Journal of Sports Medicine* 8:11–18.

Franks, B.D., and E.T. Howley. 1989. *Fitness facts: The healthy living handbook.* Champaign, Ill.: Human Kinetics.

Freid, C.R. 1983. An examination of the test characteristics of the 12 minute aerobic swim test. Master's thesis, University of Wisconsin-Madison.

Frieden, E., and H. Lipner. 1971. *Biochemical endocrinology of the vertebrates.* Englewood Cliffs, N.J.: Prentice Hall.

Galbo, H. 1983. *Hormonal and metabolic adaptation to exercise.* Stuttgart, Germany: Georg Thieme Verlag.

Galloway, J. 1984. *Galloway's book on running.* Bolinas, Calif.: Shelter Publications.

Gamberale, F. 1972. Perceived exertion, heart rate, oxygen uptake and blood lactate in different work operations. *Ergonomics* 15:545–54.

Gatti, C.J., R.J. Young, and H.L. Glad. (n.d.) Effect of water-training on the maintenance of cardiorespiratory endurance of athletes. St. Louis, Mo.: Shelter Publications.

Gavin, J. 1988. Psychological issues in exercise prescription. *Sports Medicine* 6:1–10.

Getchell, B. 1983. *Physical fitness: a way of life.* New York: John Wiley & Sons.

Gettman, L.R., M.L. Pollock, and A. Ward. 1983. Adherence to unsupervised exercise. *Physician and Sportsmedicine* 11(10):56–63.

Gibson, H., and R.H.T. Edwards. 1985. Muscular exercise and fatigue. *Sports Medicine* 2:120–32.

Gilmour, G. 1965. *Run for your life.* Sydney, Australia: Minerva Limited.

Gollnick, P.D., W.M. Bayly, and D.R. Hodgson. 1986. Exercise intensity, training, diet, and lactate concentration in muscle and blood. *Medicine and Science in Sports and Exercise* 18:334–40.

Grace, T.G. 1985. Muscle imbalance and extremity injury: A perplexing relationship. *Sports Medicine* 2:77–82.

Graves, J.E., et al. 1987. The effect of hand-held weights on the physiological responses to walking exercise. *Medicine and Science in Sports and Exercise* 19:260–65.

———. 1988. Physiological responses to walking with hand weights, wrist weights, and ankle weights. *Medicine and Science in Sports and Exercise* 20:265–71.

Gutmann, M.C., et al. 1981. Perceived exertion: Heart rate relationship during exercise testing and training in cardiac patients. *Journal of Cardiac Rehabilitation* 1:52–59.

Gwinup, G. 1987. Weight loss without dietary restriction: Efficacy of different forms of aerobic exercise. *American Journal of Sports Medicine* 15:275–79.

Hage, P. 1983. Prescribing exercise: More than just a running program. *Physician and Sportsmedicine* 11(5):123–31.

Hagerman, F.C., R.A. Lawrence, and M.C. Mansfield. 1988. A comparison of energy expenditure during rowing and cycling ergometry. *Medicine and Science in Sports and Exercise* 20:479–88.

Hagerman, F.C., et al. 1984. Muscle damage in marathon runners. *Physician and Sportsmedicine* 12(11):39–46.

Harkcom, T.M., et al. 1985. Therapeutic value of graded aerobic exercise training in rheumatoid arthritis. *Arthritis and Rheumatism* 28:32–38.

Hayden, R.M., G.J. Allen, and D.N. Camaione. 1986. Some psychological benefits resulting from involvement in an aerobic fitness program from the perspectives of participants and knowledgeable informants. *Journal of Sports Medicine* 26:67–76.

Heath, G.W., et al. 1981. A physiological comparison of young and older endurance athletes. *Journal of Applied Physiology* 51:634–40.

Henderson, J. 1969. *Long slow distance: The humane way to train.* Mountain View, Calif.: World Publications.

———. 1977. *Jog, run, race.* Mountain View, Calif.: World Publications.

Hermiston, R.T. 1967. Prediction of maximum oxygen uptake. Ph.D. dissertation, University of Michigan.

Hettinger, T. 1961. *Physiology of strength*. Springfield, Ill.: Charles C. Thomas.

Higdon, H. 1977. *Fitness after forty*. Mountain View, Calif: World Publications.

———. 1979. *On the run from dogs and people*. Chicago: Chicago Review Press.

Hill, D.W., et al. 1987. Effect of training on the rating of perceived exertion at the ventilatory threshold. *European Journal of Applied Physiology* 56:206–11.

Holloszy, J.O. 1983. Exercise, health, and aging: A need for more information. *Medicine and Science in Sports and Exercise* 15:1–5.

Horton, E.S. 1985. Metabolic aspects of exercise and weight reduction. *Medicine and Science in Sports and Exercise* 18:10–18.

Hough, T. 1902. Erographic studies in muscular soreness. *American Journal of Physiology* 7:76–92.

Howley, E.T., and M.E. Glover. 1974. The caloric costs of running and walking one mile for men and women. *Medicine and Science in Sports* 6:235–37.

Jackson, A., A.S. Jackson, and Frankiewicz. 1979. The construct and concurrent validity of a 12-minute crawl stroke swim as a field test of swimming endurance. *Research Quarterly* 50:641–48.

Johannessen, S., et al. 1980. High-frequency, moderate-intensity training in sedentary middle-aged women. *Physician and Sportsmedicine* 14(5):99–102.

Johnson, B.L., et al. 1977. Comparison of oxygen uptake and heart rate during exercises on land and in water. *Physical Therapy* 57:273–78.

Johnson, C.H., and J.W. Hastings. 1986. The elusive mechanism of the circadian clock. *American Scientist* 74:29–36.

Jonas, S., and P. Radetsky. 1986. *Pacewalking*. 3rd ed. New York: Crown Publishers.

Jones, R.D., and S. Weinhouse. 1979. Running as self therapy. *Journal of Sports Medicine* 19:397–404.

Kasch, F.W., J.P. Wallace, and S.P. Van Camp. 1985. Effects of 18 years of endurance exercise on the physical work capacity of older men. *Journal of Cardiac Rahabilitation* 5:308–12.

Katch, F.I., et al. 1984. Effects of sit up exercise training on adipose cell size and adiposity. *Research Quarterly for Exercise and Sport* 55:242–47.

Katch, V., et al. 1978. Validity of the relative percent concept for equating training intensity. *European Journal of Applied Physiology* 39:219–27.

Katz, J. 1981. *Swimming for total fitness.* Garden City, N.Y.: Doubleday.

Kirby, R.L., et al. 1984. Oxygen consumption during exercise in a heated pool. *Archives of Physical Medicine and Rehabilitation* 65:21–23.

Kline, G.M., et al. 1987. Estimation of VO_{2max} from a one-mile track walk, gender, age, and body weight. *Medicine and Science in Sports and Exercise* 19:253–59.

Knuttgen, H.G. 1986. Quantifying exercise performance with SI units. *Physician and Sportsmedicine* 14(12):157–61.

Kohrt, W.M., et al. 1987. Physiological responses of triathletes to maximal swimming, cycling, and running. *Medicine and Science in Sports and Exercise* 19:51–55.

Krebs, P.S., S. Zinkgraf, and S.J. Virgilio. 1986. Predicting competitive bicycling performance with training and physiological variables. *Journal of Sports Medicine* 26:323–30.

Kuntzleman, C.T. 1980. *Rating the exercises.* New York: Penguin Press.

Lentner, C., ed. 1981. *Geigy scientific tables.* Vol 1. West Caldwell, N.J.: Ciba-Geigy Corp.

Loftin, M., et al. 1986. Influence of physiological function and perceptual effort on 1.5 miles performance in college women. *Journal of Sports Medicine* 26:214–18.

Lollgen, H., T. Graham, and G. Sjogaard. 1980. Muscle metabolites, force, and perceived exertion bicycling at varying pedal rates. *Medicine and Science in Sports and Exercise* 12:345–51.

Long, B.C., and C.J. Haney. 1986. Enhancing physical activity in sedentary women: Information, locus of control, and attitudes. *Journal of Sport Psychology* 8:8–24.

Luce, G.G. 1971. *Biological rhythms in human and animal physiology.* New York: Dover Publications.

Lydiard, A. 1961. *Rothmans athletic training schedule.* Auckland, New Zealand: Rothmans.

———. 1978. *Running the Lydiard way.* Auckland, New Zealand: Hodder & Stoughton.

Mader, A. 1980. The contribution of physiology to the science of coaching. Koln, West Germany: Institut fur Kreislaufforschung und Sportmedizin.

Magel, J.R., and J.A. Faulkner. 1967. Maximum oxygen uptakes of college swimmers. *Journal of Applied Physiology* 22:929–38.

Makalous, S.L., J. Araujo, and T.R. Thomas. 1988. Energy expenditure during walking with hand weights. *Physician and Sportsmedicine* 16(4):139–48.

Martin, D.E., and P.N. Coe. 1991. *Training distance runners.* Champaign, Ill.: Leisure Press.

Martin, J.E., and P.M. Dubbert. 1982. Exercise applications and promotion in behavioral medicine: Current status and future directions. *Journal of Consulting and Clinical Psychology* 50:1004–17.

Massicotte, D.R., R. Gauthier, and P. Markon. 1985. Prediction of VO2 max from running performance in children aged 10–17 years. *Journal of Sports Medicine* 25:10–17.

Matheson, G.O., et al. 1987. Stress fractures in athletes. *American Journal of Sports Medicine* 15:46–58.

Mathews, D.K., R.W. Stacy, and G.N. Hoover. 1964. *Physiology of muscular activity and exercise.* New York: Ronald Press.

Matsui, H., K. Kitamura, and M. Miyamura. 1978. Oxygen uptake and blood flow of the lower limb in maximal treadmill and bicycle exercise. *European Journal of Applied Physiology* 40:57–62.

McArdle, W.D., R.M. Glaser, and J.R. Magel. 1971. Metabolic and cardio-respiratory response during free swimming and treadmill walking. *Journal of Applied Physiology* 30:733–38.

McArdle, W.D., et al. 1976. Metabolic and cardiovascular adjustment to work in air and water at 18, 25, and 33 degrees C. *Journal of Applied Physiology* 40:85–89.

McArdle, W.D., et al. 1978. Specificity of run training on VO2 max and heart rate changes during running and swimming. *Medicine and Science in Sports* 10:16–20.

McCready, M.L., and B.C. Long. 1985. Locus of control, attitudes toward physical activity, and exercise adherence. *Journal of Sport Psychology* 7:346–59.

McCunney, R.J. 1987. Fitness, heart disease, and high-density lipoproteins: A look at the relationships. *Physician and Sportsmedicine* 15(2):67–75.

McLellan, T.M., and J.S. Skinner. 1981. The use of the aerobic threshold as a basis for training. *Canadian Journal of Applied Sport Sciences* 6(4):197–201.

Mihevic, P.M. 1983. Cardiovascular fitness and the psychophysics of perceived exertion. *Research Quarterly for Exercise and Sport* 54:239–46.

Mikhail, A. 1985. Stress: A psychophysiological conception. In *Stress and coping: An anthology*, edited by A. Monat and R.S. Lazarus. 2d ed. New York: Columbia University Press.

Miller, J.F., and B.A. Stamford. 1987. Intensity and energy cost of weighted walking vs. running for men and women. *Journal of Applied Physiology* 62:1497–1501.

Miyashita, M., et al. 1985. PWC75%HRmax: A measure of aerobic work capacity. *Sports Medicine* 2:159–64.

Monahan, T. 1986. Wheelchair athletes need special treatment–but only for injuries. *Physician and Sportsmedicine* 14(7):121–23, 128.

———. 1988. Perceived exertion: An old exercise tool finds new applications. *Physician and Sportsmedicine* 16(10):174–79.

Montoye, H.J., et al. 1983. Estimation of energy expenditure by a portable accelero-meter. *Medicine and Science in Sports and Exercise* 15:403–407.

Montpetit, R.R., L. Beauchamp, and L. Leger. 1987. Energy requirements of squash and racquetball. *Physician and Sportsmedicine* 15(8):106-109, 112.

Morgan, W.P. 1972. *Ergogenic aids and muscular performance.* New York: Academic Press.

Morgan, W.P., et al. 1976. Hypnotic perturbation of perceived exertion: Ventilatory consequences. *American Journal of Clinical Hypnosis* 18(3):182–90.

Mundal, R., J. Erikssen, and K. Rodahl. 1987. Assessment of physical activity by questionnaire and personal interview with particular reference to fitness and coronary mortality. *European Journal of Applied Physiology* 56:245–52.

Murphy, P. 1984. Chronobiology: For athletes it's a matter of time. *Physician and Sportsmedicine* 12(9):158, 162–64.

Myers, L. 1977. *Training with Cerutty.* Mountain View, Calif.: World Publications.

Nadel, E.R. 1985. Physiological adaptations to aerobic training. *American Scientist* 73:334–43.

Neely, G., et al. 1992. Comparison between the Visual Analogue Scale (VAS) and the Category Ratio Scale (CR–10) for the evaluation of leg exertion. *International Journal of Sports Medicine* 13:133–36.

Nelson, D.J., et al. 1988. Cardiac frequency and caloric cost of aerobic dancing in young women. *Research Quarterly for Exercise and Sport* 59:229–33.

Newham, D.J., D.A. Jones, and P.M. Clarkson. 1987. Repeated high-force eccentric exercise: Effects on muscle pain and damage. *Journal of Applied Physiology* 63:1381–86.

Noble, B.J. 1982. Clinical applications of perceived exertion. *Medicine and Science in Sports and Exercise* 14:406–411.

Noble, B.J., et al. 1983. A category-ratio perceived exertion scale: Relationship to blood and muscle lactates and heart rate. *Medicine and Science in Sports and Exercise* 15:523–28.

Noble, B.J., and R. Robertson. 1996. Perceived exertion. Champaign, IL: Human Kinetics.

Nokes, T.D. 1985. *Lore of running*. Oxford: Oxford University Press.

Nygaard, E., et al. 1978. Glycogen depletion pattern and lactate accumulation in leg muscles during recreational downhill skiing. *European Journal of Applied Physiology* 38:261–69.

Oldridge, N.B. 1988. Cardiac rehabilitation exercise programme: Compliance and compliance-enhancing strategies. *Sports Medicine* 6:42–55.

Oscai, L.B., and W.C. Miller. 1985. Dietary-induced severe obesity: Exercise implications. *Medicine and Science in Sports and Exercise* 18:6–9.

Paffenbarger, R.S., A.L. Wing, and R.T. Hyde. 1978. Physical activity as an index of heart attacks: Risk in college alumni. *American Journal of Epidemiology* 108:165–75.

Paffenbarger, R.S., et al. 1984. A natural history of athleticism and cardiovascular health. *JAMA* 252:491–95.

Paffenbarger, R.S., et al. 1986. Physical activity, all-cause mortality, and longevity of college alumni. *New England Journal of Medicine* 314:605–13.

Palka, M.J., and A. Rogozinski. 1986. Standards and predicted values of anaerobic threshold. *European Journal of Applied Physiology* 54:643–46.

Pandolf, K.B. 1978. Influence of local and central factors in dominating rated perceived exertion during physical work. *Perceptual and Motor Skills* 46:683–98.

———. 1982. Differentiated ratings of perceived exertion during physical exercise. *Medicine and Science in Sports and Exercise* 14:397–405.

Pandolf, K.B., et al. 1984. Differentiated ratings of perceived exertion and various physiological responses during prolonged upper and lower body exercise. *European Journal of Applied Physiology* 53:5–11.

Passmore R., and J.V.G.A. Durnin. 1955. Human energy expenditure. *Journal of Physiological Reviews* 35:801–40.

Phelps, J.R. 1987. Physical activity and health maintenance: Exactly what is known? *Western Journal of Medicine* 146:200–206.

Pollock, M.L. 1973. The quantification of endurance training programs. In *Exercise and sports sciences reviews,* edited by J.H. Wilmore. New York: Acedemic Press.

Pollock, M.L., and J.H. Wilmore. 1990. *Exercise in health and disease.* Philadelphia: W.B. Saunders..

Porcari, J., et al. 1987. Is fast walking an adequate aerobic training stimulus for 30- to 69-year-old men and women? *Physician and Sportsmedicine* 15(2):119–29.

Potiron-Josse, M. 1983. Comparison of 3 protocols of determination of direct VO2max amongst 12 sportsmen. *Journal of Sports Medicine* 23:429–35.

Prochaska, J.O. 1991. Assessing how people change. *Cancer* 67:805–7.

———. 1995. Why we behave the way we do. *Canadian Journal of Cardiology* 11(Suppl A):20A–25A.

Prochaska, J.O., C.C. DiClemente, and J.C. Norcross. 1992. In search of how people change: Applications to addictive behavior. *American Pyschologist* 47:1102–14.

Pugh, L.G.C.E. 1967. Athletes at altitude. *Journal of Physiology* 192:619–46.

Reilly, T., G. Robinson, and D.S. Minors. 1984. Some circulatory responses to exercise at different times of day. *Medicine and Science in Sports and Exercise* 16:477–82.

Rifkin, J. 1980. *Entropy.* New York: Viking Press.

Rippe, J.M. 1989. *Fit for success.* Englewood Cliffs, N.J.: Prentice Hall.

Rippe, J.M., and A. Ward. 1989. *The Rockport walking program.* Englewood Cliffs, N.J.: Prentice Hall.

Robertson, R.J. 1982. Central signals of perceived exertion during dynamic exercise. *Medicine and Science in Sports and Exercise* 14:390–96.

Robertson, R.J., et al. 1986. Effect of blood pH on peripheral and central signals of perceived exertion. *Medicine and Science in Sports and Exercise* 18:114–22.

Rose, K.J. 1989. *The body in time.* New York: John Wiley & Sons.

Rosenthal, S.H. 1987. Sex over 40 . New York: St. Martin's Press.

Rosenstein, A.H. 1987. The benefits of health maintenance. *Physician and Sportsmedicine* 15(4):57–68.

Rosiello, R.A., D.A. Mahler, and J.L. Ward. 1987. Cardiovascular responses to rowing. *Medicine and Science in Sports and Exercise* 19:239–45.

Ross, R.M., and A.S. Jackson. 1990. *Exercise concepts, calculations and computer applications*. Carmel, Ind.: Benchmark Press.

Roy, S.P., and R. Irvin. 1980. *Sports medicine: Prevention, evaluation, management and rehabilitation*. Englewood Cliffs, N.J.: Prentice Hall.

Ruhling, R.O., and T.W. Storer. 1980. A simple, accurate technique for determining work rate (watts) on the treadmill. *Journal of Sports Medicine* 20:387–89.

Rusko, H., and C. Bosco. 1987. Metabolic response of endurance athletes to training with added load. *European Journal of Applied Physiology* 56:412–18.

Ryan, A.J., et al. 1983. Overtraining of athletes: A roundtable discussion. *Physician and Sports Medicine* 11(8):93–110.

Sargeant, A.J., and P. Dolan. 1987. Effect of prior exercise on maximal short-term power output in humans. *Journal of Applied Physiology* 63:1475–80.

Sears, B. 1995. *The zone: A dietary roadmap*. New York: Regan Books, HarperCollins.

Selye, H. 1937. Studies on adaptation. *Endocrinology* 21(2):169–88.

———. 1952. *The story of the adaptation syndrome*. Montreal: Acta.

———. 1956. *The stress of life*. New York: McGraw-Hill.

———. 1964. *From dreams to discovery*. New York: McGraw-Hill.

———. 1973. The evolution of the stress concept. *American Scientist* 61:692–99.

———. 1985. History and present status of the stress concept. In *Stress and coping: An anthology*, edited by A. Monat and R.S. Lazarus. 2d ed. New York: Columbia University Press.

Serfass, R.C., and S.G. Gerberich. 1984. Exercise for optimal health: Strategies and motivational considerations. *Preventive Medicine* 13:79–99.

Sheehan, G.A. 1983. *Dr. Sheehan on fitness*. New York: Simon & Schuster.

———. 1989. *Personal best*. Emmaus, Pa.: Rodale Press.

Sheldahl, L.M. 1985. Special ergometric techniques and weight reduction. *Medicine and Science in Sports and Exercise*

18:25–30.

Shellock, F.G. 1983. Physiological benefits of warm-up. *Physician and Sportsmedicine* 11(10):134–39.

Shephard, R.J. 1980. What can the applied physiologist predict from his data? *Journal of Sports Medicine* 20:297–308.

———. 1985. The impact of exercise upon medical costs. *Sports Medicine* 2:133–43.

———. 1985. Motivation: The key to fitness compliance. *Physician and Sportsmedicine* 13(7):88–101.

———. 1985. Some limitations of exercise testing. *Journal of Sports Medicine* 25:40–48.

Shephard, R.J., et al. 1987. Exercise compliance of elderly volunteers. *Journal of Sports Medicine* 27:410–18.

Sherman, W.M., et al. 1984. Effect of a 42.2-km footrace and subsequent rest or exercise on muscular strength and work capacity. *Journal of Applied Physiology* 57:1668–73.

Shneidman, N.N. 1978. *The Soviet road to Olympus.* Toronto: Ontario Institute for Studies in Education.

Simpkins, J., and J.I. Williams. 1993. *Advanced human biology.* London: Collins Educational.

Sjøstrom, M., J. Friden, and B. Ekblom. 1982. Fine structural details of human muscle fibres after fibre type specific glycogen depletion. *Histochemistry* 76:425–38.

Smith, H.K., R.R. Montpetit, and H. Perrault. 1988. The aerobic demand of backstroke swimming, and its relation to body size, stroke technique, and performance. *European Journal of Applied Physiology* 58:182–88.

Smith, J.F., and P.A. Bishop. 1988. Rebounding exercise: Are the training effects sufficient for cardiorespiratory fitness? *Sports Medicine* 5:6–10.

Smutok, M.A., G.S. Skrinar, and K.B. Pandolf. 1980. Exercise intensity: Subjective regulation by perceived exertion. *Archives of Physical Medicine and Rehabilitation* 61:569–74.

Solis, K., et al. 1988. Aerobic requirements for and heart rate responses to variations in rope jumping techniques. *Physician and Sportsmedicine* 16(3):121–28.

Sparks, K., and G. Bjorklund. 1984. *Long distance runner's guide to training and racing.* Englewood Cliffs, N.J.: Prentice Hall.

Sparling, P.B., and K.J. Cureton. 1983. Biological determinants of the sex difference in 12-minute run performance. *Medicine and Science in Sports and Exercise* 15:218–23.

Squires, R.W., et al. 1982. Effect of pro-pranolol on perceived exertion soon after myocardial revascularization surgery. *Medicine and Science in Sports and Exercise* 14:276–80.

Stainsby, W.N. 1986. Biochemical and physiological bases for lactate production. *Medicine and Science in Sports and Exercise* 18:341–43.

Stamford, B. 1987. What is exercise capacity? *Physician and Sportsmedicine* 15(4):186.

Stanish, W.D. 1984. Overuse injuries in athletes: A perspective. *Medicine and Science in Sports and Exercise* 16:1–7.

Stone, E.A. 1983. Adaptation to stress: Tyrosine hydroxylase activity and catecholamine release. *Neuroscience & Biobehavioral Reviews* 7:29–34.

———. 1983. Adaptation to stress and brain noradrenergic receptors. *Neuroscience & Biobehavioral Reviews* 7:503–9.

Sulzman, F.M. 1983. Primate circadian rhythms. *BioScience* 33:445–50.

Sutton, J.R. 1977. Effect of acute hypoxia on the hormonal response to exercise. *Journal of Applied Physiology* 42:587–92.

Sweeney, B.M. 1983. Biological clocks: An introduction. *BioScience* 33:424–25.

Tagushi, S., and S.M. Horvath. 1987. Metabolic responses to light arm and leg exercise when sitting. *European Journal of Applied Physiology* 56:53–57.

Thompson, C.E., and L.M. Wankel. 1980. The effects of perceived activity choice upon frequency of exercise behavior. *Journal of Applied Social Psychology* 10:436–43.

Tiidus, P.M., and C.D. Ianuzzo. 1983. Effects of intensity and duration of muscular exercise on delayed soreness and serum enzyme activities. *Medicine and Science in Sports and Exercise* 15:461–65.

Tokmakidis, S.P., et al. 1987. New approaches to predict VO2max and endurance from running performances. *Journal of Sports Medicine* 27:401–9.

Tremblay, A., J. Despres, and C. Bouchard. 1985. The effects of exercise-training on energy balance and adipose tissue morphology and metabolism. *Sports Medicine* 2:223–33.

Ursin, H. 1982. The search for stress makers. *Scandanavian Journal of Psychology* (Suppl. 1):165–69.

Vartebadian, R., and K. Matthews. 1990. *Nutripoints: The breakthrough point system for optimal nutrition.* New York: Harper & Row.

Velicer, W.F., et al. 1990. Relapse situations and self-efficacy: an integrated model. *Addictive Behavior* 15:271–83.

———. 1995. An empirical typology of subjects within stage of change. *Addictive Behavior* 20:299–320.

———. 1996. A criterion measurement model for health behavior change. *Addictive Behavior* 21:555–84.

Von Dobeln, W., I. Astrand, and A. Bergstrom. 1967. An analysis of age and other factors related to maximal oxygen uptake. *Journal of Applied Physiology* 22:934–38.

Wankel, L.M. 1984. Decision-making and social-support strategies for increasing exercise involvement. *Journal of Cardiac Rehabilitation* 4:124–35.

———. 1985. Personal and situational factors affecting exercise involvement: The importance of enjoyment. *Research Quarterly for Exercise and Sport* 56:275–82.

Wankel, L.M., J.K. Yardley, and J. Graham. 1985. The effects of motivational interventions upon the exercise adherence of high and low self-motivated adults. *Canadian Journal of Applied Sport Sciences* 10(3):147–56.

Wasserman, K., W.L. Beaver, and B.J. Whipp. 1986. Mechanisms and patterns of blood lactate increase during exercise in man. *Medicine and Science in Sports and Exercise* 18:344–52.

Webb, P. 1985. Direct calorimetry and the energetics of exercise and weight loss. *Medicine and Science in Sports and Exercise* 18:3–5.

Webb, P., et al. 1988. The work of walking: A calorimetric study. *Medicine and Science in Sports and Exercise* 20:331–37.

White, J.A., A.H. Ismail, and G.D. Bottoms. 1976. Effect of physical fitness on the adrenocortical response to exercise stress. *Medicine and Science in Sports and Exercise* 8:113–18.

Williams, M.H. 1988. *Nutrition for fitness and sport.* Dubuque, Iowa: William C. Brown, Publishers.

Wilmore, J.H. 1983. Body composition in sport and exercise: Directions for future research. *Medicine and Science in Sports and Exercise* 15:21–31.

———. 1986. *Sensible fitness.* Champaign, Il.: Leisure Press.

Wilmore, J.H., and D.L. Costill. 1994. *Physiology of sport and exercise.* Champaign, Ill.: Human Kinetics.

Wilmore, J.H., et al. 1986. Ratings of perceived exertion, heart rate, and power output in predicting maximal oxygen uptake during sub-maximal cycle ergometry. *Physician and Sportsmedicine* 14(3):133–43.

Winget, C.M., C.W. DeRoahia, and D.C. Holley. 1985. Circadian rhythms and athletic performance. *Medicine and Science in Sports and Exercise* 17:498–516.

Yeh, M.P., et al. 1983. "Anaerobic threshold": Problems of determination and validation. *Journal of Applied Physiology* 44:1178–86.

Young, K., and C.T.M. Davies. 1984. Effect of diet on human muscle weakness following prolonged exercise. *European Journal of Applied Physiology* 53:81–85.

Zarrugh, M.Y., and C.W. Radcliffe. 1978. Predicting metabolic cost of level walking. *European Journal of Applied Physiology* 38:215–23.

≡ ACKNOWLEDGMENTS ≡

We are all just part of a whole. Without help, much less is accomplished. Thanks to:

The many people along the way who touched this effort, but because of space, will not be mentioned personally.

The professionals—Dr. Stan James, athlete and orthopedic surgeon, who is always willing to talk about training concepts and treat the athletes I coach, and who taught me that many situations can be improved by applying "tincture of time." Dr. Gary Klug, my doctoral advisor, who allowed me to pursue my interests, and Dr. Britton Chance who invited me to work in his lab at Penn. Covert Bailey, who saw value in the L.E.A.P. concept and added suggestions that significantly improved the book. Dr. Laura VanHarn, who has continually supported and encouraged L.E.A.P. Todd Silverstein my editor at ReganBooks whose advice and persistence has significantly shaped this book. John Miller, Courthouse Athletic Clubs, Salem, Oregon, who has to be one of the best club managers in the country, for his vision, encouragement, and support. Jon and Gene Joseph, owners, Pacific Nautilus Gym and Aerobics, Eugene, Oregon, and their staff, who make a health club exactly what it should be: fun, friendly, and focused, without a lot of frills.

The businesspeople—John Beaulieu, of the Oregon Resource and Technology Development Fund, Larry Raicht, Alberto Salazar, Charles Shepard, Wade Bell, Rich Boggs, of THE STEP Company, and investors who contributed money, expertise, and patience to the development of the original L.E.A.P. computer program.

The athletes, past and present—Each day I learn something from each of you and always enjoy our time together.

My business partner—Dan Mayhew who has become a trusted friend, has made many suggestions to help L.E.A.P., and who always had faith in the concept. Also to his wife Bev, who encouraged him to follow his dream.

My family—Ruth, my former wife, who supported my pursuit of educational and coaching opportunities which resulted in the L.E.A.P. concept. Jennifer, my daughter, the best of sounding boards, who has always been on target and has never worried about how her observations would affect my feelings. We all need someone like that in our lives. Her husband Ron, who used the L.E.A.P. principles to run his first race, a marathon in 3:11:07. Steve, my son, who used the L.E.A.P. computer program and provided valuable suggestions, who convinced me I had to start writing, who proofread the versions, and who allowed me to use his poem in Chapter 17. And especially Marlene, my love and my partner for 10 years, for her beautiful sense of humor, for her patience in bearing with the trials of bringing a concept and a book to fruition, for not taking either of us too seriously, and for making it so easy to be together.